Step by Step
Phaco
Tips and Tricks
(Highlighting Woodcutter's Nucleus Cracking Technique)

Step by Step Phaco Tips and Tricks

Dr Vikas Mahatma
Ophthalmologist
Founder Medical Director
Mahatme Eye Bank and Eye Hospital
Recognised Institute for Post Graduation
Nagpur and Mumbai, India

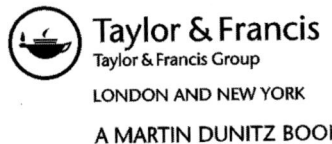

Taylor & Francis
Taylor & Francis Group

LONDON AND NEW YORK

A MARTIN DUNITZ BOOK

PGC: WW 260 MAH
KHN

© 2005 Vikas Mahatme

First published in India in 2005
Jaypee Brothers Medical Publishers (P) Ltd, New Delhi, India.
EMCA House, 23/23B Ansari Road, Daryaganj, New Delhi 110 002, India
Phones: 23272143, 23272703, 23282021, 23245672 m\, Fax: +91-011-23276490
e-mail: jpmedpub@del2.vsnl.net.in, Visit our website: www.jaypeebrothers.com

First published by Martin Dunitz, a member of the Taylor & Francis Group plc in 2005. Exclusively
distributed worldwide (excluding the Indian Subcontinent) by Martin Dunitz, a member of the Taylor &
Francis Group plc.

Tel.:   +44 (0) 1235 828600
Fax.:   +44 (0) 1235 829000
E-mail: info@dunitz.co.uk
Website: http://www.dunitz.co.uk

A CIP record for this book is available from the British Library.

ISBN 1 84184 548 5

Distributed in North and South America by

Taylor & Francis
2000 NW Corporate Blvd
Boca Raton, FL 33431, USA

Within Continental USA
Tel.: 800 272 7737; Fax.: 800 374 3401
Outside Continental USA
Tel.: 561 994 0555; Fax.: 561 361 6018
E-mail: orders@crcpress.com

Distributed in the rest of the world (excluding the Indian Subcontinent) by
Thomson Publishing Services
Cheriton House
North Way
Andover, Hampshire SP10 5BE, UK
Tel.:   +44 (0)1264 332424
E-mail: salesorder.tandf@thomsonpublishingservices.co.uk

to

My Parents .....

My Father
who inspired me
to dream of an Eye Institute
to serve the mankind

and

My Mother
who taught me to love my patients and use my
hands for manual works which helped me in
grooming my surgical skill.

My Patients .....
who complained about their postoperative
problems and taught me to improve my surgical
results continuously.

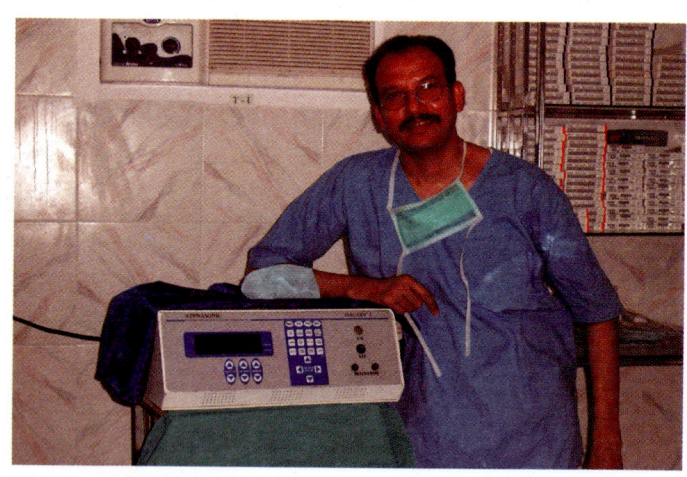

My Best Friend since the time I started Phaco!
(Author Dr Vikas Mahatme with Galaxy Appasamy
Indian made Phaco Machine)

FACES THAT GAVE A FACELIFT TO THE OPHTHALMOLOGY IN INDIA. I SALUTE THEM

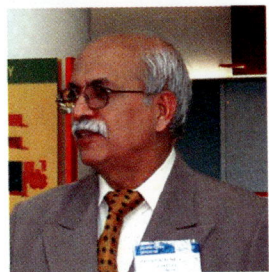

Dr Pran Nagpal

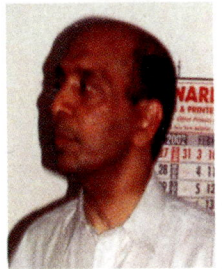

Dr GN Rao

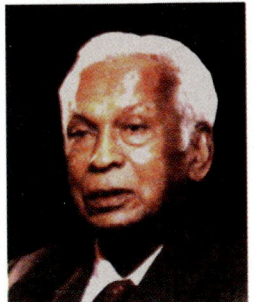

Dr G Vankataswamy

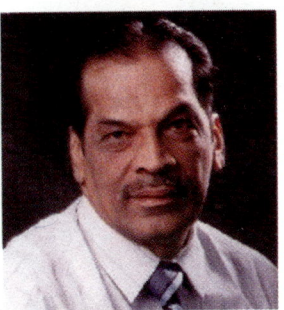

Dr Namperumal

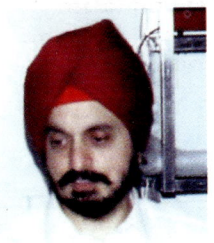

Dr HS Dua

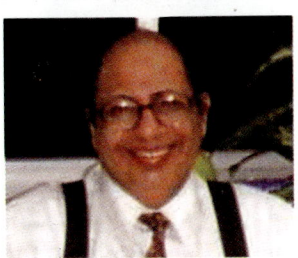

Dr Keiki R Mehta

Contd...

Contd...

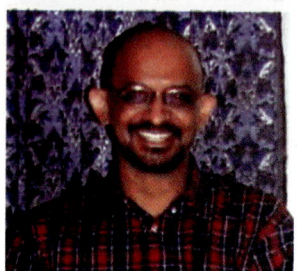

Dr Ravi Thomas

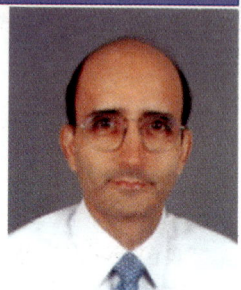

Dr Abhay Vasavada

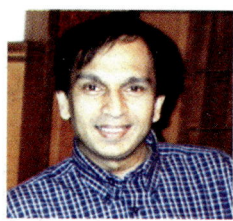

Dr Amar Agarwal

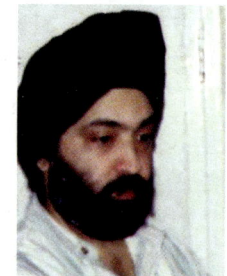

Dr Mahipal Sachdev

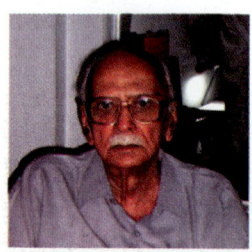

Dr Ishwarchandra

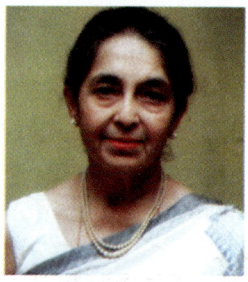

Dr Sudha Sutaria

...And there are many more ophthalmologists who have equally contributed for upliftment of ophthalmology in India. We regret our inability to provide their photographs, although they will always remain in our hearts forever.

Preface

Friends,

Way back in my residency, one of my patients had vitreous haemorrhage. I advised him Crooke's collosol iodine. He came to me after 15 days with a smile on his face. He was happy to have an improved vision. I was feeling proud about myself as I was convinced that his vision improved because of my treatment. Then I asked him, "how many times did you take that mixture?" Surprisingly, he said, "I didn't take it. I followed the instructions on the bottle. It said—"keep the bottle tightly closed!"

Then I realized that most of the times nature takes the care and surgeon catalyses the process so as to get good results. This is the reason, Phaco cataract surgery appears to me as most natural, since it does not disturb the nature gifted anatomy of eye to a great extent.

Over the years, Phacoemulsification is no longer the latest technology but undoubtedly the excellent, time-tested way of cataract surgery. Unfortunately, many new surgeons don't allow this technology to enter their minds. The most possible reason being fear and apprehension of learning new technique and a scare of causing harm to the patients while learning. But friends, I too wasn't an exception to this fear. I have passed through every stage of it, realising later, how unjustified my thoughts were prior to learning phaco. I am also aware of the feelings of a phaco learner—his problems and his worries. This is the reason I thought of bringing out this handy book dealing with very practical and vital aspects of phacoemulsification.

This book has been written with the aim of giving practical tips for developing surgical skill. It does not contain the facts that are well established beyond doubts and are given in details in several text books. The theme of the book revolves round the concept "**we have to learn how to learn**". This is especially true for surgical techniques where we want to learn but without compromising the vision of patient. This has been stressed all through this book. After phaco many new techniques may arrive but this book will be like a Bible that will take away your fear of learning and adapting the new technique because now you know the proper path of mastering any new procedure. I have elaborated about actions to be taken when we do not get desired results at any surgical step.

As my experience grew, one of my patients said, "doctor you have good skill and I bless you that your skill helps all the patients." First I thought, he is talking something that is impossible. On a second thought, I realised that this can be made at least partly possible, if I am able to transfer my skills through this book.

I shall like to acknowledge the persistence of my wife Dr. Sunita. Like any wife she was nagging me but this time for a good constructive cause of getting this book completed by me. My goals are her goals. If I say I want to write a book, she will create environment to write the book. Although professionally she is a gynecologist, by heart she is an ophthalmologist. She has helped me in many ways and by all means to improve the quality of this book.

There are many more whose names I might not have written here they are like foundation of a building which remains invisible; they have directly or indirectly helped me in completing this book. Also last but not the least, the residents and fellows who came here to learn phaco, also shared their problems with me, which they came across while learning phaco. This has added to my experience.

Friends, once I asked my son Chinmay, "what is your dream?" He said, "I want to live in a developed country". I was shocked! I asked him further, "in which country?" He said *"DEVELOPED INDIA"*! Friends, let us equip ourselves against blindness with new weapons like phacoemulsification. Let us make our contributions to convert developing India into developed India. Let us help in making the dreams of upcoming generation become true and make them live happily with good vision in a developed India.

Thanks.

Vikas Mahatme

Why Should I Read This Book?

Friends,

In 1993 I was attending American Academy's meeting at Chicago, when the phacoemulsification had just made its way and someone asked me if I would like to go in for Phaco. Being an established private practitioner, doing lot of work with small incision extracapsular cataract extraction, my answer was a strong 'No'. A couple of years later I found myself converted into a Phaco surgeon. Today the situation is such that cataract surgery is almost synonymous with phaco. I am not exaggerating, but almost every day a new book on phacoemulsification is coming up. Then why read this book?

The aim behind publishing this book is to share my journey towards Phaco, my views, my experiences, and the problems I faced in the subject. I am sure, they will be beneficial for all those who are still in dilemma of whether to go in for Phaco or not, for those who want to learn how to start and also for those who are already doing Phaco. You will find in this book, **concepts converted into practical tips** and guidelines, rather than mere theory. These are extremely important as far as mastering the technique is concerned. At the same time, you may feel that some important points are missing from this book. I have avoided them because they are well established and accepted facts, which can be read from a textbook on Phaco.

Just as you cannot learn swimming by reading a book on 'How to Swim' you can not learn any surgical procedure, unless you start doing it. So, get started; start doing Phaco; refer to the guidelines as and when required. Whenever you are in problem, refer to this book again. I am sure; phacoemulsification will soon be a friendly affair for you.

Why Should I Shift to Phaco?

Whatever may be your ophthalmic specialty; you are bound to encounter a patient of cataract, because it still remains the commonest problem. So, why not adopt the latest in the field; especially when changing over to latest is beneficial to the patient as well as to surgeon?

Remember there was a storm in 1980s, when it was time to change over from intracapsular lens extraction to extracapsular lens extraction with intraocular lens implantation. The question then was, "Why shift over to extracapsular cataract extraction and IOL when I can give 20/20 vision with intracapsular cataract extraction and aphakic glasses thereafter? Extracapsular cataract extraction and IOL have chances of additional complications, while learning..." and so on. You know the history, how the new procedure miraculously changed the scenario for patients as well as for ophthalmologists that now we laugh at ourselves at the questions we had in minds at the time of changeover. We were afraid of complications—not of the procedure but complications during the learning phase. Later on we realized that it was not the technique that was at fault, but the problem was faulty way of learning a new technique.

Similarly, we now blame phacoemulsification for possibility of additional complications. In fact we need to master the technique by *"proper way of learning"*. If this happens we will not have to repeat the history and laugh at ourselves once again.

Whenever a new surgical technique is to be accepted and adopted it should first clear a *Three-Way test* based on scientific approach.

1. Is it better than existing procedure?
2. Is it safe?
3. Is it economically viable or feasible?

Let us apply this test to phacoemulsification and weigh its efficacy.

Is it better than existing extracapsular cataract extraction with IOL procedure?

The advantages of phacoemulsification over extracapsular cataract extraction are well known and need not be elaborated in details. In brief, one can say that it is a small incision procedure, as well as *least traumatizing*, with *no iris touch* that usually invokes inflammation. "*No Stitch, No Patch, No Injection Anesthesia*" is the selling slogan for Phaco surgery. With corneal incision it is difficult to identify the eye that has been operated next day. This is because of least inflammation it invokes as compared to manual small incision cataract surgery.

Is it safe?

When an old surgical procedure is to be compared with a new technique, it is a wrong policy to compare results of new procedure done at the hands of inexperienced novice surgeon with that of old procedure done by an experienced surgeon. Ideally, comparison should be between new and old procedures done by an expert in respective techniques. Reason is simple. As narrated earlier, learning the technique may be at fault rather than technique itself. Surgeon may land up in problem and complications, while learning any new procedure. This is the reason that *"we have to learn, how to learn"*. If this dictum is followed, it is beyond doubt that Phacoemulsification has fewer complications as compared to routine extracapsular cataract extraction. It is a procedure with a better control.

Economic Feasibility and Viability

One feels that Phacoemulsification machine itself costs a great deal and then there are recurrent expenses as well. However, once you master the technique recurrent cost is much less and even comparable to extracapsular cataract extraction. As it happens with every electronic gadget, slowly the cost of machine is bound to come down. The earlier you buy a machine, the more you might spend but be sure, the most you will be benefited because you are then a "Phaco surgeon", that distinguishes you from the crowd.

IF YOU THINK EDUCATING AND UPGRADING YOURSELF IS TIME CONSUMING AND EXPENSIVE, THEN TRY IGNORANCE!

While thinking about 'To be or not to be', some more questions crop up in our mind. These questions may take out enthusiasm to learn phaco. The questions may be like these—

1. I am working at periphery or in camps. Patients' paying capacity is much less.

Once you master the technique, more number of patients can be operated in shorter time. Patient can be discharged as in day care center. Complications are less. Patients need not come for repeated follow-up. This automatically reduces overall cost of treatment. Also it is **not mandatory to use foldable IOL**; instead, 5.2 mm diameter Phaco lenses are good enough to solve the purpose. Even foldable IOL are becoming affordable now a days as lower priced foldable IOL are coming up. **Phaco camp is no more an imagination**. We have been doing it; anybody can do it.

> IF NOT NOW THEN WHEN?
> IF NOT YOU THEN WHO?

2. I am new in practice. I don't have substantial volume of patients. Phacoemulsification is of no use to me.

A newcomer in the practice ought to have an edge over the established ophthalmologists. Then only he can make a place for himself. Then why not have with you an asset like Phaco, which can distinguish you from the lot. Remember, however, that learning should be without spoiling a single case. Patient's vision is of supreme importance. To know how to do it, you will have to go through the subsequent chapters.

3. I am an ophthalmologist of good reputation, doing significant amount of surgical work. I am happy with the results. Learning new technique will snatch away my prime time.

Learning is an investment rather than wasting time. Once you expertise, your time per case will be saved. Follow up headaches will be reduced. Ultimately phacoemulsification will be a time saver on a long run.

It seems to me that any future research in newer techniques will definitely be based on Phaco technique only. This is the reason learning phacoemulsification will soon become a basic requirement for any ophthalmic surgeon. When you are adopting Phaco, biomedical industry is with you all the time—when you buy a machine, when you have problems in learning the technique, or when you wish to update yourself by learning the latest in the field and they also help by continuously improving the machine.

YOU GET MEDALS ONLY IF YOU GO THROUGH WARS !

Contents

Converting from Extracapsular Cataract Extraction Surgeon to a Phaco Surgeon: A Stepwise Approach

Strong motivation and inclination on your part in favor of phaco is the first step and makes learning process much easier. It is as good as winning half the battle. Our motto should be, **Learn: But not at the cost of vision.** How to achieve this is our next problem. Let us deal with this problem step by step. It is funny to know that learning phacoemulsification starts much before you buy a machine. You can start learning few steps like operating from temporal side in routine extracapsular cataract extraction, capsulorhexis and hydrodissection during routine extracapsular cataract extraction procedure, which you have mastered already. Try to enlarge routine capsulorhexis of 4 or 5 mm by taking relaxing incisions at 2 and 10 o'clock with capsulotomy needle (26G needle with a bent tip) or cystitome.

With capsulotomy needle try to scratch the capsule at 2 and 10 o'clock position, from periphery to center. If this is not sufficient, do not mind taking multiple incisions at other positions, with the bent needle but always from periphery to center. With this, you can deliver out the nucleus just as you do it in canopener capsulorhexis technique. You can then continue with extracapsular cataract extraction procedure as before (refer chapter on Capsulorhexis). Next step is to learn hydrodissection. (refer chapter on Hydrodissection for details).

The moment you buy the phaco machine, you are so thrilled and elated that your fingers start itching to start doing phaco right from the very first day. Phaco machine becomes your prestigious belonging. And you want to let the whole world know about your recently purchased jewel. This is the time when you need to refrain from promoting yourself as a phaco surgeon. Remember, you are just an owner of the phaco machine and soon you are going to be a phaco master!

Avoid announcing formal inauguration of your new phaco machine till you are a confident phaco surgeon. You may put yourself in trouble if you advertise about your possession of the machine. If you let everybody know about your phaco machine, everyone will expect and may insist you to operate by phaco.

YOUR TENSE MOMENT CAN BE A SIGHT FOR OTHERS!

Your colleagues in operation room are eagerly waiting to watch you doing phaco. This is when exactly the whole problem starts. Remember that ***there is always a 'U'-turn possible from Phaco to routine extracapsular cataract extraction*** and you should never mind shifting back to extracapsular cataract extraction at any step. Between your pride and patient's vision, the winner should be patient's vision.

Your first duty is to make yourself and others in operation room aware of the fact that use of phaco machine is going to be a gradual process and will take some time.

Getting acquainted with machine is a necessary step. You have to sit with the machine and get accustomed to various audible signals. You need to train your ears about sounds produced when irrigation – aspiration is on, phaco- is on, vent mechanism is active, when preset vacuum is reached and about other parameters. You also need to take a view of preset vacuum power, actual phaco power, flow rate, phaco time and other details of machine.

Then comes the role of your feet. It is just like learning steps of a dance. Right foot has to get a judgment of pressure required to make irrigation on, aspiration on, phaco on. It is just like moving about the accelerator of your car. You should be able to recognize audible signals like vacuum reached or not and so on, without looking at the machine. Perfect tuning of ears, foot and machine can lead to a successful phaco orchestra.

Phaco involves all senses like legs, hands, eyes, ears and so on. It sounds rather difficult that we have to use multiple senses and organs at the same time. This feeling may scare you. However, don't you think that we have been trained since our childhood, to use our eyes, ears, feet, hands and mind simultaneously? Remember good old days when we were learning to ride a bicycle, a two-wheeler or even a car. Moreover learning two wheelers involves balancing too. There is always risk to the learner's life. Wasn't all this difficult at that time? See, how smoothly you can drive now. Then why be afraid of learning Phaco? At least here there is no danger of loosing our balance. In one of the phaco workshops I was conducting, someone commented that you don't loose vision while learning bicycle. But remember, while learning bicycle we have all possibilities of injuring ourselves. Still we continue learning and practicing it.

Get tuned to the machine. You should learn the meaning of different audible signals. Then, on goat's eye try doing phaco. It is difficult to learn chopping on goat's eye but you can learn fluidics. Try to maintain anterior chamber while doing phaco in goat's eye. Try to maintain the foot switch in position 2 (that is aspiration on) with preset vacuum reached. You should be able to move to position 3 (phaco on) and come back to position 2 and maintain the preset vacuum. You should be able to bring the foot switch to position zero if iris is caught. Develop all these reflexes. In brief, you should get accustomed to the foot, ear and hand coordination. According to your wish you should be able to control the foot switch. The moment you think that you need aspiration; reflexly your foot should be able to go to aspiration position of the foot switch. There is a difference in knowing about it and actually doing it reflexly. Unless you practice it several times, you can not act swiftly.

Simultaneously you have to make yourself aware about the theory of Phacodynamics. Attending workshops and conferences on phaco, visiting phaco surgeons, observing them at surgery, does help at this time.

Then we climb one more step and come to mastering main phaco incision (refer chapter on Incisions). For this you can use steel blade. First try it on goats' eyes and eye bank eyes. Once the skill is achieved, then try on patient's eye. Try making incision sitting on **'temporal side'**; assess yourself. Sitting on temporal side is advantageous as conversion to routine ECCE is very easy from 12 o'clock position. Exact site of the incision depends on whether you are operating on right eye or left eye and also on whether you are a right handed surgeon or left handed. If you are a right handed surgeon and operating on patient's right eye then incision at 12 o'clock position is alright for ECCE. However, if you are operating on patient's left eye it is better to take the incision slightly on nasal side. This is because the main phaco incision is on upper temporal side in left eye, which will come in the way of ECCE incision at 12 o'clock. *Follow the dictum of patting yourself for the good steps you have learnt and at the same time considering your areas of improvement (or your shortcomings)*. As far as this patient is concerned, your job of learning this step is over; forget about rest of the phaco surgery once you have made phaco incision; operate from superior limbus and proceed with routine extracapsular cataract extraction. Phaco incision is also a self-sealing incision which by and large does not leak. If at all it leaks, you can suture it with 10-0 polygalactin. Eye bank eyeballs are fairly good enough to learn these steps on. Never do too many new steps on single patient.

Once you feel confident of doing main phaco incision and side port incision properly, try both the steps together in next patient. While doing this, make a side port incision first and if you find it OK, then proceed with main phaco incision or else you can convert to routine extracapsular cataract extraction even after side port incision. The rule is, **"At whatever step you feel uncomfortable, convert to routine extracapsular cataract extraction"**.

You know how to make main phaco and side port incisions in one patient. It is now time for you to insert phaco handpiece and make just a light sculpt in central area. (It is assumed that you have already performed capsulorhexis and have mastered the art. This is possible before you have the phaco machine (see Capsulorhexis)). Even if you are successful in sculpting at the very first attempt, do not proceed further with next step. Your first attempt of inserting a phaco handpiece has to end here. Take a pause. It is again a time for self-assessment. Take note of your strengths and your weaknesses or area of improvement. Proceed with routine extracapsular cataract extraction operating from 12 o'clock. To proceed further with phaco especially when you are doing it correctly, is the biggest temptation to resist. Never fall prey to it. Things become easy, after you are confident of sculpting and making incisions. **Remember, patience always pays here !**

Mastering phacodynamics is always better. When anterior chamber gets collapsed, or becomes shallow, it indicates that you have to take a review of fluidics again. If anterior chamber becomes shallow at any moment, identify the problem and rectify it. (See chapter on FAQ).

Once you know, you can sculpt well, start sculpting in central nuclear part in the next patient. Make a groove in central part of nucleus. Stop. Shift back to routine extracapsular cataract extraction from 12 o'clock. After delivering out the nucleus, assess the depth of groove made by phaco handpiece on the nucleus. This gives you idea about your assessment of depth of groove while operating and the actual depth that has occurred. This kind of an assessment will let you know how much to sculpt for the required depth.

Cracking of nucleus is the next step to learn only after you have ensured mastery on previous steps (refer to chapter on Woodcutter's Technique). Its time now to shift back to extracapsular cataract extraction again.

Learn how to break nucleus into 4 pieces. Then try to complete the surgery with phaco. Posterior capsular rupture chances are there when you try to engulf **last nuclear fragment**. You have to be very cautious at this time. You should not regret any time if you think it is not possible to proceed further with phaco. You should rather feel happy that you have not compromised with patient's vision.

Hold Yourself from Doing Phaco

- When capsulorhexis is not complete.
- If irrigation fluid used is more than 250 ml, convert yourself to routine extracapsular cataract extraction.
- If linear phaco time is more than 2 min. 30 seconds. This is because if you continue you will feel comfortable and next day you may find corneal edema.
- If there is a rent in posterior capsule or you are in

dilemma whether there is a rent or not convert immediately to routine extracapsular cataract extraction.

- If at any time you are in two minds, whether to continue with phaco or not, never continue with Phaco and convert to conventional extracapsular cataract extraction.

Gradually you can master automated irrigation aspiration too. It is easier and safe to learn bimanual irrigation and aspiration. An important step is learning to release the footswitch without moving your hand whenever posterior capsule is caught in irrigation aspiration port. When posterior capsule is caught, our natural reflex is, we try to pull out the handpiece, which further leads to a rent in posterior capsule.

After mastering these **steps**, you have now become a routine Phaco surgeon. A time has now come that you have to learn doing phaco in complicated cases like— very hard nucleus, non-dilating pupil, and very shallow anterior chamber, in incomplete capsulorhexis. Then learn how to shift over to surgery under topical anesthesia (see chapter on Frequently Asked Questions). Once you have conquered these problems, you will be a master. Then you will be in a position to teach other surgeons who are Phaco beginners.

Here I shall like to enlighten you more about memory. If we know how it works, it is easy to learn any new skill. There are various ways by which memory is recorded in our brain. One of the types is *action memory*. The examples of action memory are typing, swimming, cycling and of course *performing surgery*. The more you do it, better you perform. Reading theory is important, but equally important is practicing the action and storing it in action memory. Many times in action it is difficult to explain how to do a particular thing, but it is easy to do it actually. Like when you ride a bicycle you can balance yourself but it is difficult to tell others how to do that. This can be achieved only when you practice it as many times that the action happens at a subconscious level (see chapter Actions that Speak for Themselves). This does not mean that you are supposed to practice on patients. How to learn this? We will see in coming chapters.

Once you get thorough with theoretical aspects of phacodynamics, accustomed to machine signals, foot-switch and know coordination on goat's eyeball, then you are all set to start learning on patient. It is always an asset to have with you a skilled phaco surgeon around you when performing phaco in the initial stages. This however may not be possible always, except in an institute.

STEPWISE LEARNING

Dictum: Always do one step at a time, forget about phaco and continue doing routine extracapsular cataract extraction after learning each step.

ONE WHO DOES TOO MANY THINGS ACCOMPLISHES NOTHING

PRAISE YOURSELF! REWARDED BEHAVIOUR IS REPEATED.

ECCE surgeon (extracapsular cataract extraction)
↓

[1] ECCE surgeon motivated for phaco
↓ → Buy phaco machine..... Preferably

[2] Read theory, phacodynamics, attend workshops

[3] Learn on goat's eyes → Side port incision

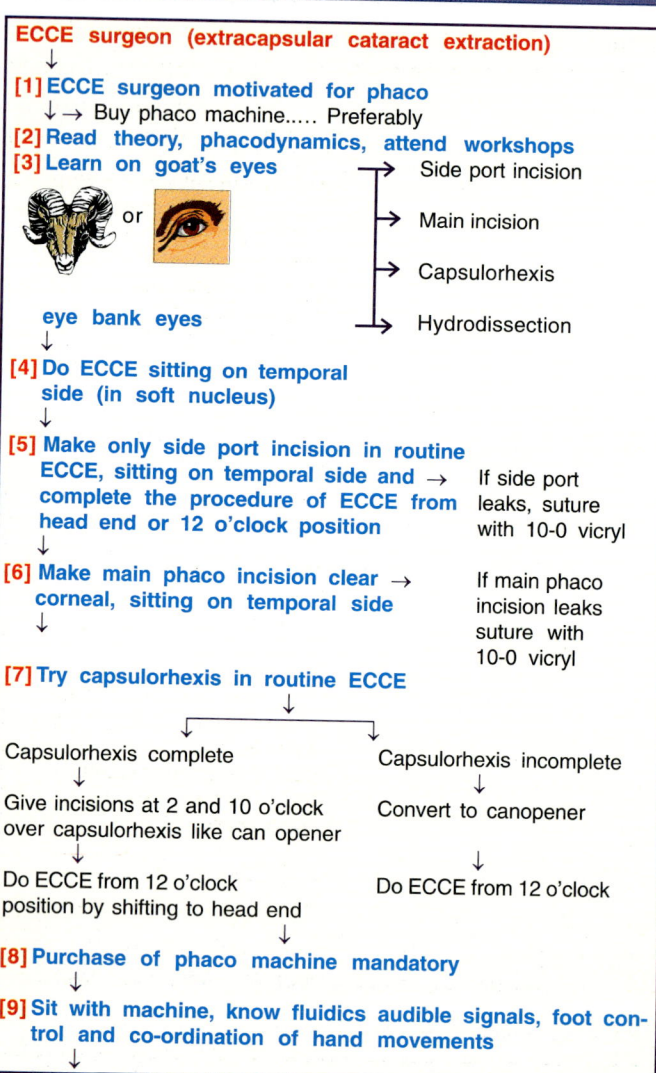

→ Main incision

→ Capsulorhexis

eye bank eyes → Hydrodissection
↓

[4] Do ECCE sitting on temporal side (in soft nucleus)
↓

[5] Make only side port incision in routine ECCE, sitting on temporal side and → If side port **complete the procedure of ECCE from** leaks, suture **head end or 12 o'clock position** with 10-0 vicryl
↓

[6] Make main phaco incision clear → If main phaco **corneal, sitting on temporal side** incision leaks suture with 10-0 vicryl
↓

[7] Try capsulorhexis in routine ECCE
↓

Capsulorhexis complete   Capsulorhexis incomplete
↓   ↓
Give incisions at 2 and 10 o'clock   Convert to canopener
over capsulorhexis like can opener
↓   ↓
Do ECCE from 12 o'clock   Do ECCE from 12 o'clock
position by shifting to head end
↓

[8] Purchase of phaco machine mandatory
↓

[9] Sit with machine, know fluidics audible signals, foot control and co-ordination of hand movements
↓

Contd...

Contd...

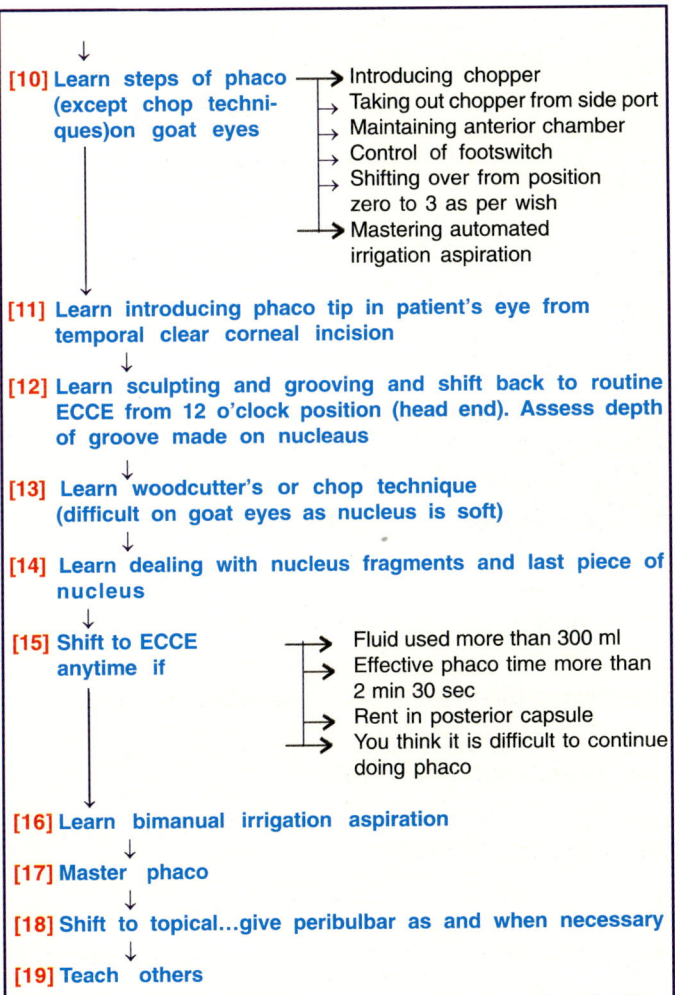

[10] **Learn steps of phaco (except chop techniques)on goat eyes** → Introducing chopper
→ Taking out chopper from side port
→ Maintaining anterior chamber
→ Control of footswitch
→ Shifting over from position zero to 3 as per wish
→ Mastering automated irrigation aspiration

[11] **Learn introducing phaco tip in patient's eye from temporal clear corneal incision**

[12] **Learn sculpting and grooving and shift back to routine ECCE from 12 o'clock position (head end). Assess depth of groove made on nucleaus**

[13] **Learn woodcutter's or chop technique (difficult on goat eyes as nucleus is soft)**

[14] **Learn dealing with nucleus fragments and last piece of nucleus**

[15] **Shift to ECCE anytime if** → Fluid used more than 300 ml
→ Effective phaco time more than 2 min 30 sec
→ Rent in posterior capsule
→ You think it is difficult to continue doing phaco

[16] **Learn bimanual irrigation aspiration**

[17] **Master phaco**

[18] **Shift to topical...give peribulbar as and when necessary**

[19] **Teach others**

Flow Chart 1.1: Key to learning phaco stepwise

If you take a review of all these steps for learning you will come to know approximately after how many patients you will be able to perform your first phaco surgery completely. This will help you to learn patiently. **Haste never Helps.** Actually the learning curve is not so long, if you go stepwise. Do not worry; you are definitely going to make optimum use of your phaco machine because very soon you are going to be an excellent phaco surgeon. Pat yourself after every new step, you have learnt successfully. Take a note of your strengths and weaknesses; concentrate on areas of improvement.

> ### HAVE A LION'S HEART! LOOK BACK AFTER YOU HAVE WALKED FEW STEPS.

1. The whole chain of events starts when a surgeon, who is well versed with Extracapsular Cataract Extraction, gets motivated to go in for phaco. Outwardly you are the same person for others. But from inside you know that you are different and better as you are motivated for phaco and soon you will be a good phaco surgeon.

2. The moment this happens, you should start reading about theory part and attend as many workshops as possible. Though not mandatory at this stage, it is preferable to buy a phaco machine for this itself creates a strong force for learning phaco. The reason is very simple; you do not want to see your machine

lying idle. (Your banker will remind you every month that you have to learn phaco)!

3. On goat's eye or eye bank eyes start learning
   a. Side port incision
   b. Main phaco incision
   c. Capsulorhexis
   d. Hydrodissection.

4. Now sitting on temporal side, try extracapsular cataract extraction in soft nuclei, so that you get accustomed to operating from temporal side and also to the hand rest and posture. But initially choose cases with soft nuclei, as it is easier to do.

5. Next step is to do side port incision by sitting on the temporal side in routine extracapsular cataract extraction preferably when eye to be operated is left and if you are a right handed surgeon. This is because the side port incision will not come in your field of operation as it will be towards 6 o'clock position. Once this is done, move again to head end and carry on with routine extracapsular cataract extraction. The patient in whom you are learning side port incision, try to do only this step, from temporal side, forget rest of the phaco procedure and shift over to extracapsular cataract extraction again from superior limbus. Do not try to make major incision in the same patient. Side port incision may or may not leak. If side port incision is not up to the mark or shows leak, suture it with 10-0 Polygalactin. If it does not leak then forget the incision it seals on its own.

6. Similarly try to do main phaco incision clear corneal (why clear corneal? See chapter on Incisions) and sitting on the temporal side in routine ECCE. This is especially easy in right eye surgery and the surgeon is right handed. As the main phaco incision is in lower half of cornea it will not come in way of routine ECCE. Once you finish doing main phaco incision, shift back to head end (12 o'clock position) and complete the procedure by ECCE. If this incision leaks suture with 10-0 polygalactin. If it does not leak then forget it. The incision will seal on it's own.

7. Then try capsulorhexis in routine extracapsular cataract extraction. Sitting on temporal side make main phaco incision and try capsulorhexis with forceps.

   a. If capsulorhexis is complete and satisfactory, try hydrodissection. Give cuts at 10 and 12 o'clock positions and do extracapsular cataract extraction while sitting at 12 o'clock position (head end of patient).

   b. If capsulorhexis is incomplete, convert to can opener. Shift to head end side and complete the procedure by routine extracapsular cataract extraction.

8. The time has now come when buying a phaco machine is mandatory now.

9. Spend some time sitting with the machine, getting acquainted with fluidics, audible signals, foot control, hand and feet coordination and so on. Doesn't

it sound like you have fallen in love and dating a friend?

10. Try to do phaco in goat's eyeball. Remember that it is difficult to do phaco in goat's eyeball, as the nucleus is very soft. So what can we learn in goat's eye?
    a. To introduce chopper and take out chopper from side port.
    b. Learn to maintain anterior chamber always deep while operating. You learn fluidics. To maintain anterior chamber means to control footswitch.
    c. To shift over from position zero to 3 whenever you wish. Learn to know the audible signals at different levels. Like irrigation on, irrigation and aspiration on. Signal of preset vacuum achieved etc.
    d. To master automated irrigation aspiration. This trains you to maintain anterior chamber and learn fluidics.
11. In patient's eye make clear corneal temporal incision and introduce phaco tip through it.
12. Make sculpting and then grooving. Shift again to head end and complete the procedure by routine extracapsular cataract extraction. After removing nucleus out examine it and assess the depth of groove. This gives you idea about exact pressure you have to exert for sculpting in your next patients. Depth of groove you have made.
13. Learn chop technique or woodcutter's technique. This step is difficult to be learnt on goat's eyeball as

the nucleus is very soft. This problem can be overcome by—

a. Replacing nucleus of goat's eyeball by nucleus removed from patient who has undergone ECCE. In our institute we do it in a special way. Whenever patient is operated by ECCE, we store this nucleus in deep refrigerator (freezer). Then in goat's eye phaco incision is taken, capsulorhexis is done and then incision is enlarged to put the frozen ECCE nucleus in the capsular bag. This incision is now sutured again. Thereafter the eye is rotated to make fresh incision for the phaco handpiece and learn cracking the nucleus.

b. Using eye bank eyes with iris removed from it. For this also we, at our institute, have developed our own technique. We take whole eyeball from eye bank. The corneal epithelium is removed by scraping. A main phaco incision is made and iris is removed from it with forceps. The capsule is then stained with trypan blue, rhexis is done and then nucleus-cracking technique is learnt.

14. Learn dealing with nucleus fragments and last piece of nucleus.

15. Switch over to routine extracapsular cataract extraction from head end if,

a. Fluid used is more than 250 ml. There is always a temptation to continue surgery but next day you will find corneal edema.

    b. Effective phaco time exceeds 2 minutes and 30 seconds.

    c. Whenever you are in dilemma whether to continue phaco or not, then do not continue. Convert to extracapsular cataract extraction.

    d. Even If you suspect least that there might have been a rent in posterior capsule.

16. Learn bimanual irrigation aspiration.

17. Master phaco by practicing.

18. Shift to topical. Here comes again a warning. Do not make it a prestige issue. Whenever needed, supplement with peribulbar block. Its very easy to shift over to block at any moment as this is a closed chamber surgery and incisions are self-sealing. One can push viscoelastics inside the anterior chamber and give massage over eyeball. One need not be afraid of high vitreous pressure.

19. Teach others. We always forget that some day we were also a student who needed a helping hand. What if nobody guided us then? Teaching others is like re-paying the loan! This will help in keeping alive and growing the breed of phaco surgeons!

EACH ONE OF US NEEDS A HELPING HAND TO GROW. ONCE GROWN, GIVE YOURS.

Chapter 2

Capsulorhexis

You can learn capsulorhexis—a vital step in phaco surgery even before purchasing a phaco machine. Capsulorhexis is like a window to learn phaco. Doing phaco is possible in a canopener capsulorhexis too, but you need to be an expert phaco surgeon to do this. A phaco learner should never try phaco when capsulorhexis is incomplete. In that case it is better to convert to extracapsular cataract extraction. This is the reason learning capsulorhexis forms one of the fundamental essentials for phaco beginner. Capsulorhexis is like a gateway to the world of phaco.

One of the prerequisites of a capsulorhexis is flat anterior capsule, which in other words means a deep anterior chamber. There are two ways to learn capsulorhexis, either with a capsulotomy needle or with forceps. You can try it by piercing cornea 1 mm inside limbus, at any comfortable position using 26 G bent needle (capsulotomy needle). This, you can try first in routine extracapsular cataract extraction before opening anterior chamber. Needle will have a 2 cc syringe containing hydroxypropyl methylcellulose attached to it. Less viscous hydroxypropyl methylcellulose only can come out through 26 G needle; otherwise you can use normal saline. Always aim at a smaller capsulorhexis for it is easy to enlarge it afterwards (refer Enlarging capsulorhexis).

You can learn (see below How to Learn) capsulorhexis with forceps if you practice doing this on goat's eye. You can do it well on patients eye if a clear corneal self-sealing incision is taken. (In that case hydroxypropyl methyl-cellulose will not come out easily). An added advantage of clear corneal incision is that approach is direct and maneuver of instruments in anterior chamber is easy as compared to that in scleral self-sealing incision. With routine extracapsular cataract extraction, if you try to do capsulorhexis through scleral incision then anterior chamber collapses. This is because the incision is not self-sealing. In this case it is better to do needle capsulorhexis before opening anterior chamber as stated in previous paragraph. For capsulorhexis with forceps it is better to take self-sealing phaco incision. The incision width may be 2 mm to start with. The small width of incision is beneficial, as Hydroxypropyl methylcellulose does not come out from the anterior chamber. The Utrata-Inamura forceps can be used through small incision too. As compared to utrata forceps, this Utrata-Inamura forceps has more firm grip and better control. Capsulorhexis with forceps specially Utrata-Inamura is easier, takes less time and more controlled procedure as compared to capsulorhexis done by needle. This is my personal experience. I think this is because additional force in upward direction can be applied with forceps.

What to do if capsulorhexis is extending towards periphery

Always try to maintain a deep anterior chamber. The direction of tip of the capsular flap of capsulorhexis should be on the side in which you want to drag it out (Fig. 2.1) the grip of the forceps or the force of the needle should be near to the base of the flap.

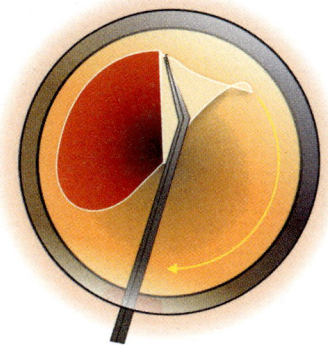

Fig. 2.1: The direction of the flap should be on the same side to which you want to drag it, in such a way that the flap falls on itself

Utrata-Inamura capsulorhexis forceps can hold a good chunk of capsular flap and has good leverage. Therefore it is easier to draw the capsular tag towards center than with Utrata forceps which can catch hold of only a tiny portion of tag and hence we can not control its dragging. Remember the direction of pull should always be towards center and towards posterior capsule when you want to pull the capsulorhexis margin in.

It is always preferred to hold the inner as well as outer surface of the capsule rather than only the outer surface especially when the capsulorhexis is extending towards periphery (Fig. 2.2).

The capsulorhexis, that has extended towards periphery, you may feel is difficult to be brought to the center. This is because zonules try to stretch the capsule towards

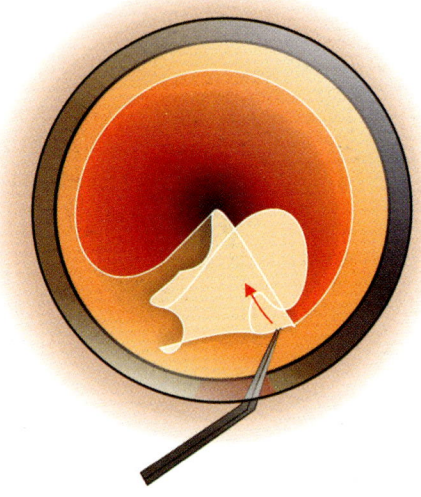

Fig. 2.2: The margin is extending to the periphery; hold the inner as well as outer surface of the capsular flap

periphery. This results in tendency for the capsular tear to extend to the periphery. This also results in false impression. You feel that capsulorhexis, that has extended to the periphery, is 1 or 2 mm inside when in reality it is 1 or 2 mm away towards periphery (Fig. 2.3). In reality it is not difficult to bring back the capsulorhexis, which has extended towards periphery, if, we understand the above forces.

If it has extended towards periphery then hold the base of flap with Inamura-Utrata forceps and hold it as mentioned in previous paragraph. Then pull the flap towards the center and posteriorly, instead of pulling it anteriorly, towards the cornea and center. This is because

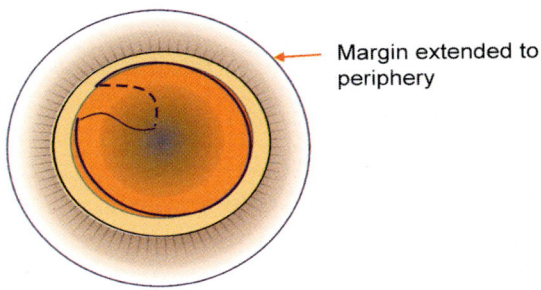

Fig. 2.3: The margin actually has not been extended to the periphery though we feel as if it has been extended to the periphery

of zonules which stretch the capsule towards periphery and anteriorly (Fig. 2.4). This force is neutralized by the pull towards posterior capsule and center. So in all cases it is possible to complete the capsulorhexis even if it has gone towards periphery. If capsulorhexis extends beyond

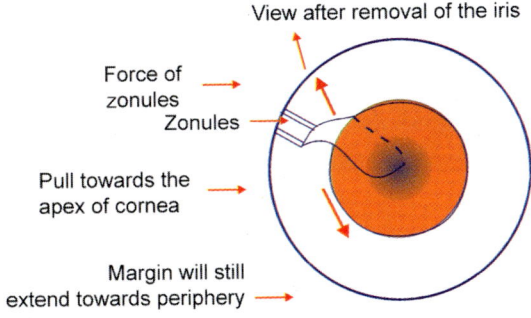

Fig. 2.4: This figure shows the force of zonules on the capsule. If we try to pull the rhexis margin towards the apex of the cornea, both the forces pull the anterior capsule in different direction, thus further extending the tear towards the periphery

7 mm, zonules try to stretch the capsular tag towards periphery. In this situation, if we don't take note of this fact then we may have to end up with incomplete capsulorhexis.

If capsulorhexis is extending towards periphery, hold the capsule with Inamura-Utrata forceps in such a way that one of the tongs holds the flap of capsule from inside and another from outside. If possible pull should be towards posterior capsule (downwards) and not towards cornea (Fig. 2.5).

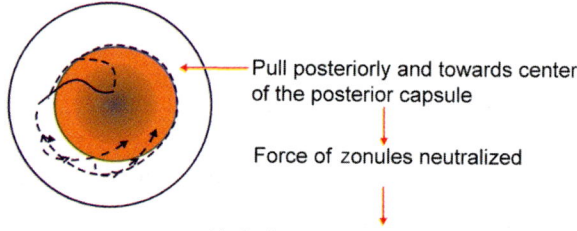

Pull posteriorly and towards center of the posterior capsule

Force of zonules neutralized

No further extension towards priphery

Fig. 2.5: This figure shows exactly how the pull should be there, that is towards the center of posterior capsule

TO TRY AND FAIL IS OKAY BUT TO FAIL TO TRY IS TRULY TRAGIC

Capsulorhexis in Hypermature Cataract

There are two major problems with hypermature cataract:
1. Poor visibility of capsular flap.
2. Extension of capsular flap towards periphery.

To deal with poor visibility, put some methylcellulose drops over cornea. This acts like a convex lens and improves visibility temporarily by magnifying view without compromising with field of vision. You also need to take out cortical fluid intermittently with the help of hydroxypropyl methylcellulose by repeatedly injecting it and taking it out.

Use of **Trypan blue** is a great boon today. I inject hydroxypropyl methylcellulose using a cannula having an opening at top (Fig. 2.6) since the direction of the opening is facing upwards, methylcellulose coats the endothelium, which offers some protection to it. While injecting trypan blue, I keep the opening of cannula facing the capsule. (See Fig. 2.7, showing opening of the cannula and hydroxypropyl methylcellulose and trypan blue coming out through it). Layer of methylcellulose over corneal endothelium prevents trypan blue from coming in contact with it. At the same time we achieve desired action of Trypan blue, i.e. staining of the capsule so that it becomes clearly visible against white background.

To prevent the problem of extension of capsulorhexis towards periphery, anterior chamber should always be kept deep (by injecting hydroxypropyl methylcellulose). First nick on anterior capsule should be large enough so that the intralenticular fluid comes out easily. The small nick means small opening in the capsule. If this happens and if the intralenticular pressure of fluid is more, intralenticular fluid tries to come out with force in anterior chamber. This causes extension of small capsular opening and tear extends towards periphery (Figs 2.8A to C). The question is how to avoid that small nick? When you make the first nick there should be at least 3 mm distance in the

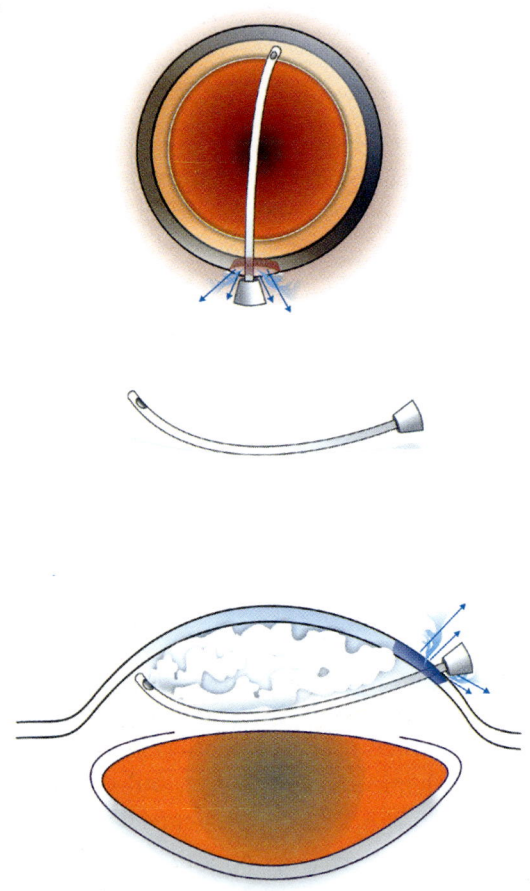

Fig. 2.6: The direction of the opening of cannula faces towards the endothelium for hydroxypropyl methylcellulose

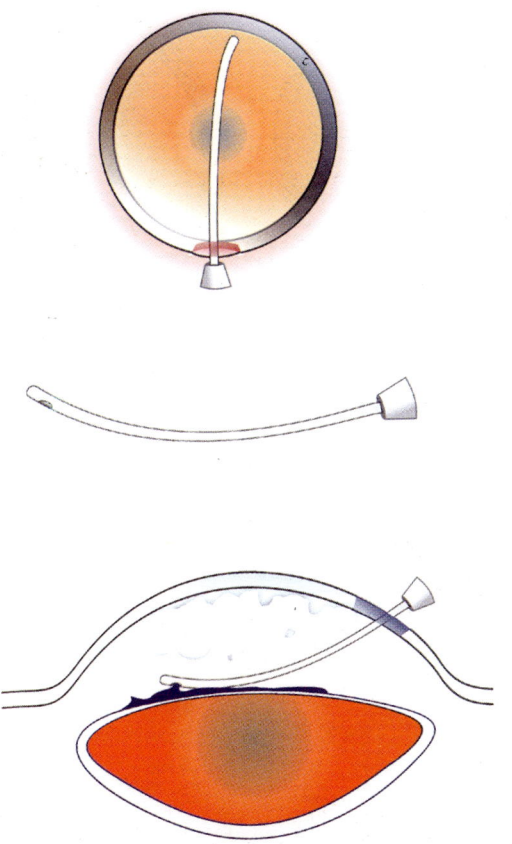

Fig. 2.7: The direction of the opening of this cannula faces towards the anterior capsule. Trypan blue is just smeared over the anterior capsule with cannula, avoiding corneal endothelium

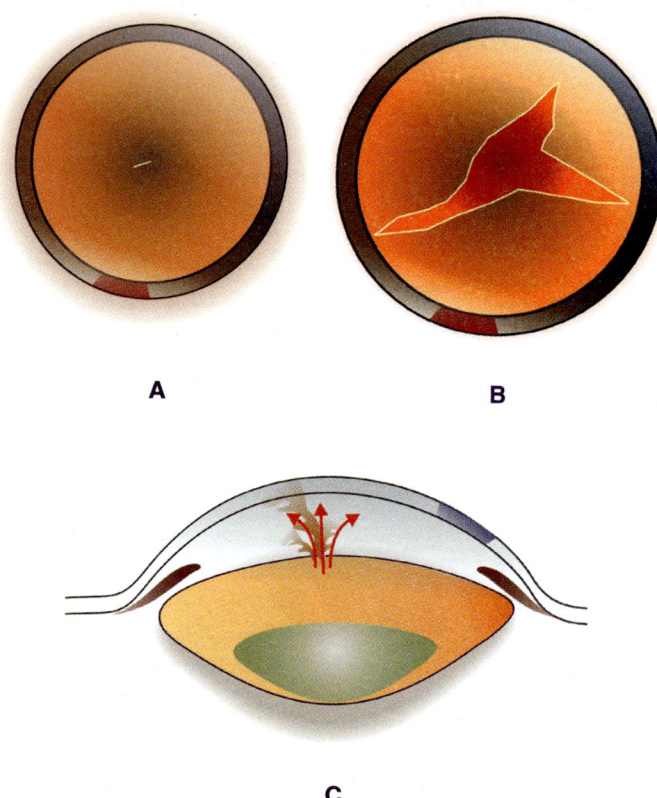

A B

C

Figs 2.8 A to C: Small nick is given over the anterior capsule. Such a small nick may extend towards the periphery. **B.** This figure shows how the nick has been extended towards the periphery. **C.** High intralenticular pressure forcing the cortex outside which causes sudden extension of the rhexis margin to the periphery

two prongs of capsule holding forceps. This helps in making a large opening in the capsule, intralenticular fluid comes out easily and rest of the problems is taken care of automatically (Figs 2.9 and 2.10).

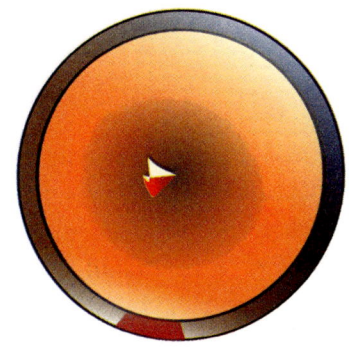

Fig. 2.9: Shows large triangular nick

Fig. 2.10: Shows high intralenticular pressure forcing the cortex outside but because of larger nick the rhexis does not extend to the periphery

Try to restrict size of the capsulorhexis to 3 or 4 mm approximately. For this Inamura-Utrata forceps is beneficial. After completing small rhexis, aspirate out all cortical matter with automated irrigation and aspiration. Push hydroxy-propyl methylcellulose in anterior chamber, enlarge the capsulorhexis and then proceed with phaco.

How to Enlarge Capsulorhexis?

To do this anterior chamber should be filled with methylcellulose. Capsule is cut with capsule cutting scissors. Giving a small nick in a concentric manner or circular fashion does this (Fig. 2.11). Hold capsular flap with capsular forceps (better with the Inamura-Utrata) and enlarge the capsulorhexis. The flap should be pulled in the direction of posterior capsule. Giving the nick in concentric manner prevents extension of rhexis to the

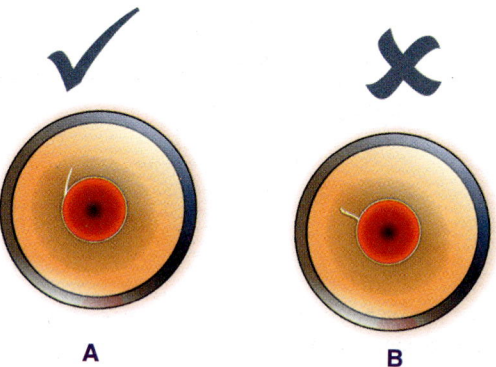

A   **B**

Figs 2.11A and B: A. While enlarging the capsulorhexis a small nick is given in concentric manner. **B.** Straight horizontal nick should be avoided

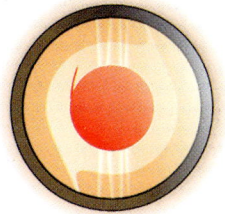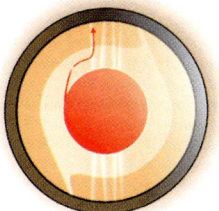

Fig. 2.12: If the loop of haptic lies near the cut of the capsulorhexis then there are more chances of extension of the capsulorhexis to the periphery. Therefore one should be cautious and place haptic away from capsular nick

periphery. If intraocular lens is already in the bag, be cautious at the sites where loops are present. At this place capsule is slightly stretched and there is increased possibility of extending capsular nick to the periphery (Fig. 2.12). I have mentioned the steps to avoid extension of rhexis to periphery in earlier paragraphs.

How to do phaco when capsulorhexis is incomplete or it has extended towards periphery?

Here, the basic aim is to avoid further tearing off or an extension of anterior capsulorhexis towards posterior side. This is achieved by:

1. Maintaining anterior chamber deep throughout procedure. The moment you take phaco handpiece out, anterior chamber collapses. To avoid this, push methylcellulose from side port incision so that anterior chamber remains deep and maintained and is never shallow. Then only take the phaco handpiece out.

2. Avoiding stretch on capsule especially at the site of capsular tear.
   a. During chopping do it 90 degrees away from site of extension of incomplete capsulorhexis.
3. While doing phaco, the nuclear fragments should not pull the capsular tear towards corneal side. This extends the capsular tear towards periphery.

Size of Capsulorhexis: Does it matter?

- It is easier to do smaller rhexis but it is difficult to do phaco with small rhexis. It is very easy to do phaco in large rhexis, but large rhexis is difficult to perform, as while doing capsulorhexis there are high chances that it may extend to periphery.

- In small rhexis, the maneuverability is difficult. For example, to place chopper and phaco tip you get very little space and then division of nucleus becomes difficult.

- Hydrodissection is difficult if rhexis is very small. The fluid does not come out easily. The path the fluid has to cross is long and sometimes it may raise intra-lenticular pressure and rupture of posterior capsule (Fig. 2.13).

- It is better to perform larger rhexis in hard cataract so that division of nucleus is easier.

- If rhexis is very large and if rent in posterior capsule occurs, it is difficult to place IOL in ciliary sulcus, as there is less support of anterior capsule.

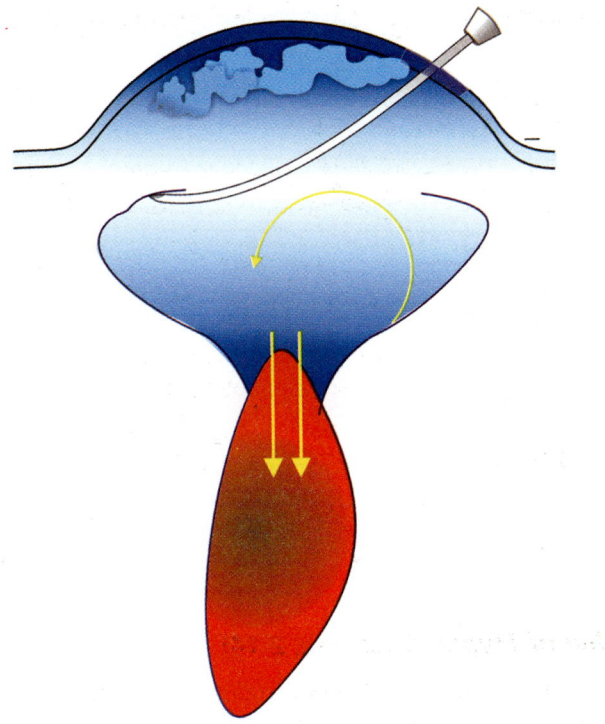

Fig. 2.13: High intralenticular pressure caused during hydro-dissection, leading to posterior capsular rupture and nucleus drop

- In very young patients and in hypermature morgagnian cataract, always aim at a very small rhexis.
- 5 to 6 mm rhexis is ideal in most of the cases.

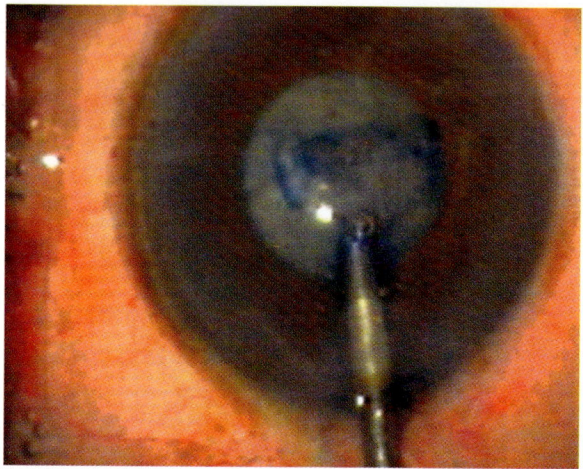

Fig. 2.14: Shows spreading of the trypan blue over anterior capsule

How to learn capsulorhexis?

Use of Trypan Blue (Fig. 2.14)

In our institution, we use Trypan blue in all cases for beginners and during phaco training programs. This has distinct advantage that while doing phaco you can see the capsulorhexis border very clearly.

How to use it?

See page No. 31, Fig. 2.7.

Advantages

1. To identify the anterior capsule in mature and hypermature cataracts. In such type of cataracts you

do not have a red glow and thus, staining of anterior capsule helps in identifying it.

2. In case your microscope is not that good, and you are not able to see a good red glow, in such case, it is very helpful if, you stain the anterior capsule with trypan blue and then do the capsulorhexis.

3. In all cases for beginners it is better to inject an air bubble in the anterior chamber and then inject trypan blue. If visco is injected instead of air then it becomes little difficult for the trypan blue to spread over the anterior capsule and stain it.

Disadvantages

1. If more trypan blue is injected it may hamper the red glow by making everything bluish.

2. It is supposed to be toxic to the corneal endothelium capsulorhexis can be learnt best on goats' eye. In my opinion, Inamura-Utrata forceps is best instrument to use for capsulorhexis. This instrument can open up even if incision is small. Because of this the viscoelastics will not come out through incision while doing capsulorhexis. Secondly, the grip of capsule is firmer as large chunk of capsule tag is in the grip as compared to other instrument. This helps in better control of capsulorhexis (Fig. 2.15).

I have observed that phaco fellows in our institute find it easier to do it with forceps as compared to needle capsulorhexis. This may be because there is an additional forces available in upward direction that is missing in case of needle capsulorhexis.

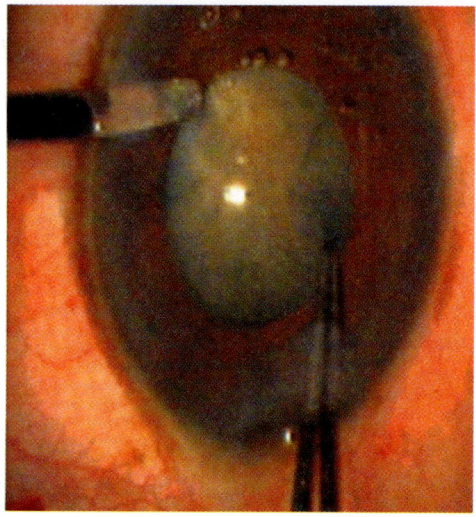

Fig. 2.15: Shows how the capsular flap is held
by the forceps while doing capsulorhexis

Once you master the art on goat's eye you can start
doing on patients eye in routine extracapsular cases. There
are two options that are possible. If you fail, convert it to
can opener. If you succeed then give relaxing incisions at
10 and 2 o'clock position on capsule. This will help to
deliver nucleus for conventional extracapsular cataract
extraction, since it is difficult to take out nucleus through
intact capsulorhexis of 5-6 mm.

Chapter 3

Hydrodissection and Hydrodelineation

Like capsulorhexis, hydrodissection also can be learnt before you are in possession of a phaco machine. It is second step to be mastered after capsulorhexis.

In hydrodissection we aim to separate cortical matter from capsular bag so that rotating nucleus and cortical aspiration becomes easy (Fig. 3.1).

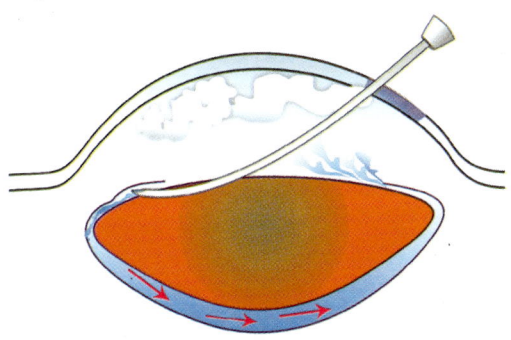

Fig. 3.1: Separation of the cortical material from capsular bag

Principles and Prerequisites of Hydrodissection

1. Fill the anterior chamber with hydroxypropyl methyl-cellulose but take care that it should not become too deep. It is better that it is little bit shallow.

2. Whatever amount of fluid enters anterior chamber should come out from incision site. If fluid does not come out through incision site, it will press over nucleus, causing sudden rupture of posterior capsule. This leads to sinking of nucleus in the vitreous. **Most of the time nucleus drop is because of faulty hydro-dissection procedure rather than Phaco itself.**

3. Do hydrodissection always through main Phaco incision, and not through side port incision. Because sometimes the fluid will not come out and increase the intralenticular pressure causing rupture of posterior capsule and nucleus drop (Fig. 3.2).

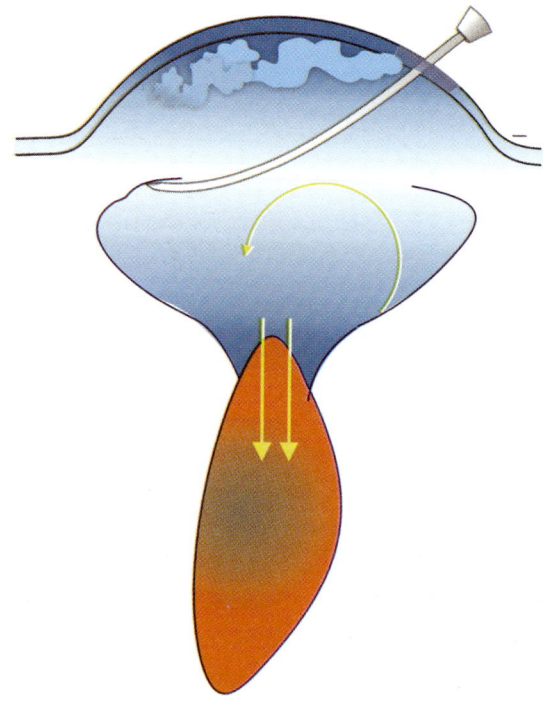

Fig. 3.2: Nucleus drop because of high intralenticular pressure

4. While doing hydrodissection, **press over posterior lip of incision, with hydrodissection cannula,** so that fluid can come out easily (Fig. 3.3).

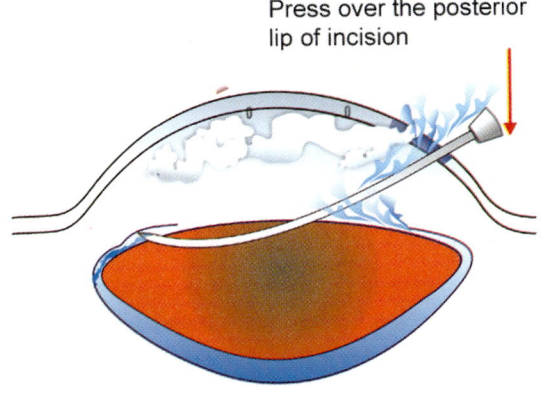

Press over the posterior lip of incision

Fig. 3.3: Shows how the pressure is given on the posterior lip of incision with hydrodissection cannula itself

5. Keep in mind that when there is a way out for the fluid to come out then only fluid can be pushed in easily. So to press over the posterior lip of the incision is very important.

6. Incision should not get closed with prolapsed iris. This will not allow the fluid to come out. This happens especially in hypermetropic eyes and eyes with non-dilating pupil. Take care while doing hydrodissection in these patients (Fig. 3.4).

7. Every time if you want to repeat hydrodissection or inject more amount of fluid then tap over the nucleus so that the fluid collected behind the nucleus comes out.

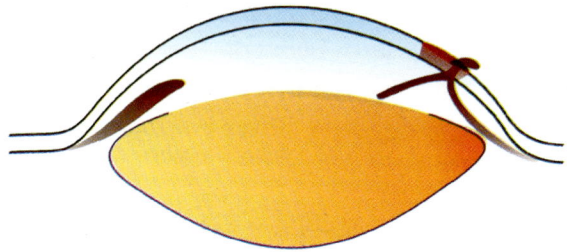

Fig. 3.4: Shows iris prolapse through the main incision. This is mostly because of the incision which is more on the limbal side

Procedure

Inject hydroxypropyl methylcellulose in anterior chamber keeping the chamber slightly shallow. (This helps fluid to come out).

Hydrodissection is done with a hydrodissection cannula, which is fixed to a 2 ml syringe containing irrigating fluid—either normal saline or ringer lactate. The quantity of irrigating fluid should never be more than 1.5 ml. If it is more, pressure on the plunger is uneven. Fluid coming out will not have smooth flow. Introduce hydrodissection cannula in the anterior chamber through main phaco incision. Lift up the edge of anterior capsule with cannula. Routine teaching advocates going up to the equator (i.e. periphery of capsular bag). Contrary to this I recommend staying away from periphery. Push 0.2 to 0.5 ml of irrigating fluid, pressing nucleus little bit with same hydro-dissection cannula and at the same time pressing on the posterior lip of the incision. The main phaco incision should be open while doing the hydrodissection (Fig. 3.5).

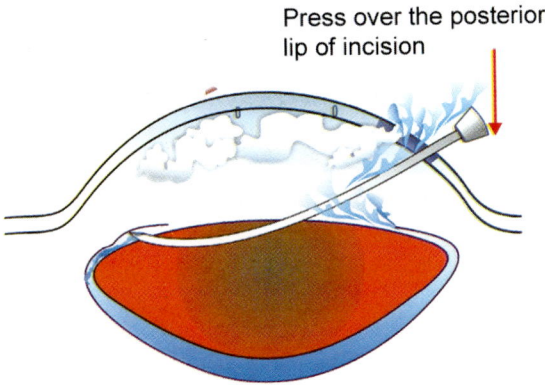

Press over the posterior lip of incision

Fig. 3.5: Shows how the pressure is given on the posterior lip of incision with hydrodissection cannula itself

You can judge completion of hydrodissection by seeing a wave of fluid passing beyond the nucleus against the red glow. Another indicator of completion of hydro-dissection is that anterior chamber becomes shallow. If you are sure that the procedure is complete, push methylcellulose in anterior chamber. This will deepen anterior chamber. Then proceed further. Try to rotate nucleus with the help of Sinsky hook or a lens dialer preferably from side port so that anterior chamber remains deep and there is no stretch over the zonules. In learning phase if we do it from main incision then there are chances of hydroxypropyl methylcellulose coming out and anterior chamber becoming shallow. If anterior chamber becomes shallow and still rotation of nucleus is tried then it stretches the zonules. So it is better to deepen the anterior chamber and then rotate the nucleus (Fig. 3.6).

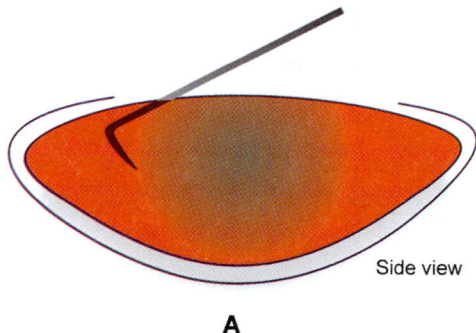

Side view

A

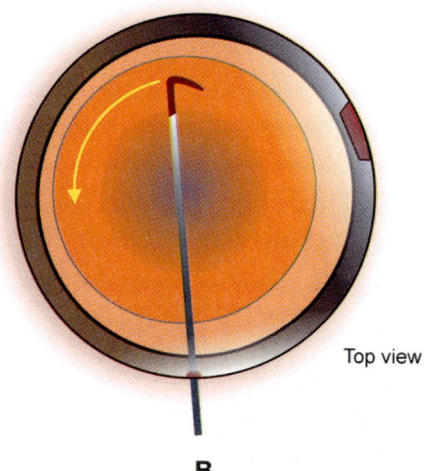

Top view

B

Fig. 3.6: Shows how the nucleus has been rotated. The anterior chamber should be kept deep while rotating the nucleus

When nucleus is very soft, with the routine Sinsky hook it is not possible to rotate the nucleus. You can try to rotate it with a Mushroom dialer. This has small ball tip so it does not penetrate the soft nucleus. This can rotate the nucleus.

During rotation of nucleus anterior chamber should be maintained deep. This avoids stretch on zonules. Sometimes, rotation of nucleus is not possible. In such case you can repeat hydrodissection. After repeating hydrodissection also if you are unable to rotate nucleus, make a groove in the center of the nucleus with Phaco. Then repeat hydrodissection. This facilitates fluid coming out from capsular bag.

Is it necessary to do hydrodissection at multiple sites?

Routinely it is not needed. In an incomplete hydro-dissection, however, you can try at other sites. Easiest is to do at a site opposite to main Phaco incision.

When Hydrodissection should not be done?

In cases with a weak posterior capsule, as in congenital or developmental cataract and posterior polar cataracts, hydrodissection should be avoided. Most of time these patients present themselves at the age of 20 to 40. If we examine these patients on slit lamp there is onion pearl like cataractous changes (Plaque cataract). In these patients hydrodissection should be avoided. In these cases there is always a possibility of posterior capsule rupture because of hydrodissection. Instead of hydrodissection, you should go for hydrodelineation in these cases.

If you are learning hydrodissection before buying a machine, i.e. during routine extracapsular cataract extraction, it is better to learn hydrodissection in central curvilinear capsulorhexis and not in can opener capsulotomy. This is because if it is done with incomplete capsulorhexis then the hydrodissection may cause extension of the capsular tear posteriorly. You should avoid pushing more than 0.5 ml of irrigating fluid. At the same time take care that anterior chamber doesn't collapse completely.

How to learn Hydrodissection?

1. Try it in goat's eye more than ten times.
2. Once you have mastered the main Phaco incision from temporal side (read chapter 1) and capsulorhexis is performed then try doing hydrodissection as per steps explained above. After this you can do routine ECCE from head end side (see chapter 1).

HYDRODELINEATION

The aim is to separate nucleus from epinucleus and cortex (Figs 3.7A to C). The advantage of this procedure is that even if anterior chamber collapses during phaco, the probability of touch of the tip to the capsule will be less. The epinucleus and cortex will act as a cushion between the tip and capsule. This offers you some safety against rent in posterior capsule by phaco tip touch. Hydro-

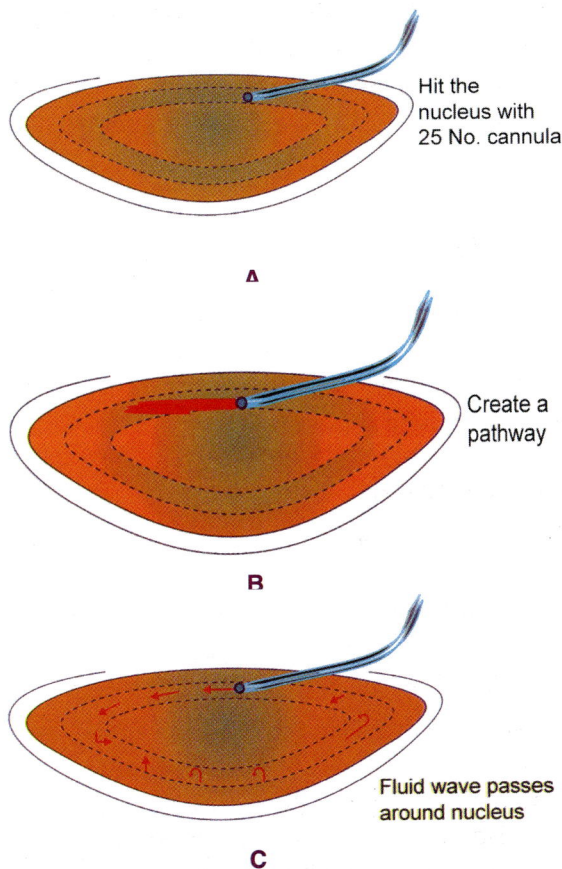

Figs 3.7A to C: A. Hit the nucleus with cannula. **B.** Create a pathway for fluid. **C.** The nucleus has been separated from the epinucleus

delineation is not required in all the cases. In the learning phase of Phaco it is preferable to do hydrodelineation in all cases. Once you master the technique of phaco-emulsification, hydrodelineation is not necessary. It is then indicated especially when hydrodissection is not possible as in weak posterior capsule or posterior polar cataract.

How and why nucleus drop occurs?

In routine ECCE we were not aware of any nucleus drop complication. Then why it occurs in phaco?

Let us see why it occurs

Suppose you are doing hydrodissection, while doing hydrodissection, you are pushing the fluid but it is not coming out. Then gradually pressure in anterior chamber shall increase. This presses over the lens and posterior capsule. If the pressure is increased to a great extent then it may cause rupture of posterior capsule resulting in dislocation of the lens in vitreous. This mishap never occurs in routine extracapsular cataract extraction, because the pressure in anterior chamber is never more than vitreous pressure. However, this can occur in any closed chamber surgery, like manual, small incision cataract surgery; especially during hydrodissection (Fig. 3.8).

The basic patho-physiology of this problem is either tremendously high pressure in anterior chamber with a weak posterior capsule or increased intralenticular pressure with a normal posterior capsule.

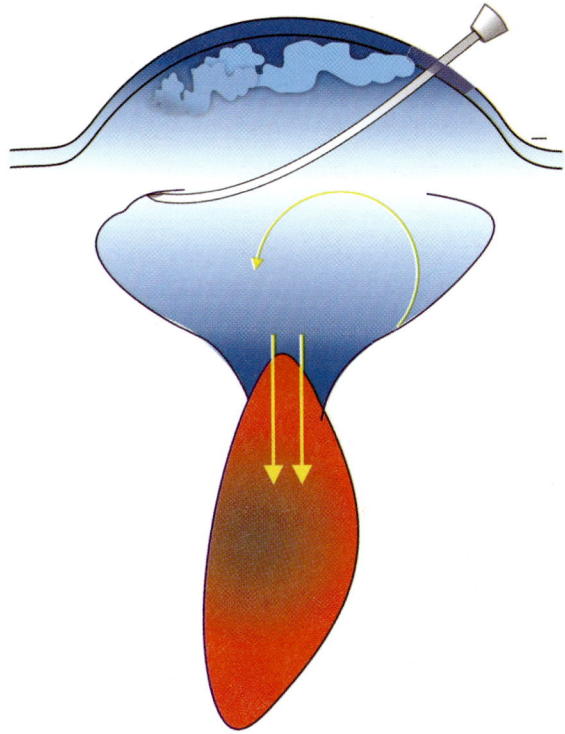

Fig. 3.8: Shows drop of the nucleus following
hydrodissection in close chamber

Imagine a situation. You have noticed a rent in
posterior capsule. Still you are continuing with Phaco. Here
also the increased pressure in anterior chamber will push
the nucleus fragment posteriorly, if it is not adherent to
cortical matter or vitreous band.

How to face this mishap—dislocation of lens in the vitreous or lens drop—to know this, please refer to page no. 131, 132.

How to avoid nucleus drop?

We have seen how nucleus drop occurs. (Refer page no. 52). The best way to tackle it is to prevent it. The challenge now is how to avoid a nucleus drop?

a. Avoid doing hydrodissection where you anticipate a weak posterior capsule as in posterior capsular cataract with onion pearl opacity or patient aged 40 years or less. (Refer Fig. 8.6).

b. While doing hydrodissection, see to it that amount of irrigating fluid entering inside anterior chamber should nearly equal the amount of fluid coming out. In this way, IOP in anterior chamber never increases. Avoid doing hydrodissection from side port read chapter on Hydrodissection .

c. While doing hydrodissection from main incision, always press over the lower flap of incision, so that fluid can easily come out.

d. Problem of raised pressure in anterior chamber to a great extent is encountered in shallow anterior chamber, hypermetropic eyes and eyes with semi-dilated or constricted pupil. One has to be very careful and vigilant in these cases. After injecting 0.5 ml of irrigating fluid, tap the nucleus so that fluid comes out.

e. Sometimes iris itself may block incision site. This will prevent outflow of the fluid from anterior chamber; avoid this.

f. Fluid should be injected slowly and not more than 0.5 ml at one time. If anterior chamber becomes shallow, one should stop injecting. Give a tap over the nucleus and take out the fluid. This, anterior chamber becomes slightly deep. Now again inject the fluid if necessary.

FOUR CHOICES OF DEALING WITH FRUSTRATION:
1. ACCEPT IT
2. RESENT IT
3. INVENT A SOLUTION
4. PREVENT IT

Chapter 4

Incisions

It is advisable to learn side port incision before main phaco incision.

Side Port Incision: How to Learn?

It is possible to learn side port incision before buying a phaco machine, initially on goat's eyeball or eye bank eyes and then in routine extracapsular cataract extraction. The side port incision should be square shaped, i.e. length, breadth and depth of incision being equal. It should be around 1 mm or less (Fig. 4.1). It is easier to do this using a 20 G needle to which a syringe, containing methyl-cellulose, is attached. The bevel of needle should be facing iris preferably. Choose the site on left side of main incision used for extracapsular cataract extraction. This is for right-handed surgeon. Incision should be 0.5 mm inside the limbus in routine cases. If anterior chamber is shallow or

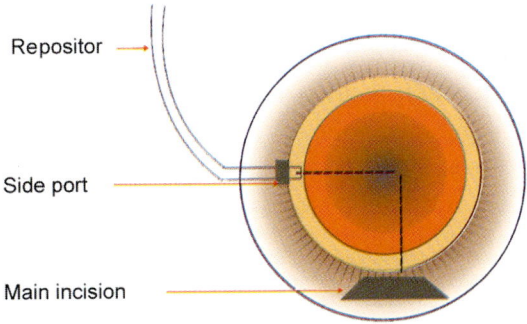

Repositor

Side port

Main incision

Fig. 4.1: Shows the approximate size of the side port and main incision

if you are aiming at small capsulorhexis, it should be 1 mm. inside the limbus. Advantage of taking incision more towards the center is that maneuverability of chopper as well as aspiration of subincisional cortical matter from side port are easy (Fig. 4.2). When you are making a side port incision, try to support the eyeball from opposite clock position at limbus by a swab stick. Never use forceps in place of swab stick, because it is very painful under topical anesthesia. Advantage of 20 G needle over other routine surgical blades is that if anterior chamber starts collapsing, you can push methylcellulose and maintain anterior chamber through the same needle. This is not possible with routine blades. Another thing is that sharpness of needle is constant in every needle (so you know how much pressure you need to exert every time) and of course, the needle is disposable, affordable.

Incision is stretched with needle as compared to MVR blade but then the advantage is that maneuverability is better. Second advantage is less amount leakage. This is because the needle incision has very small flap. This wraps around the chopper. So leakage is less and maneuverability is better. Secondly the hydration of incision does not occur easily. One can use 20 gauge MVR blades instead of needle.

While pushing hydroxypropyl methylcellulose, take care that eyeball is not too tense, which has an additional danger of optic nerve atrophy, because high pressure will cause central retinal artery occlusion. Pressure inside should be slightly higher than normal IOP, but not very high.

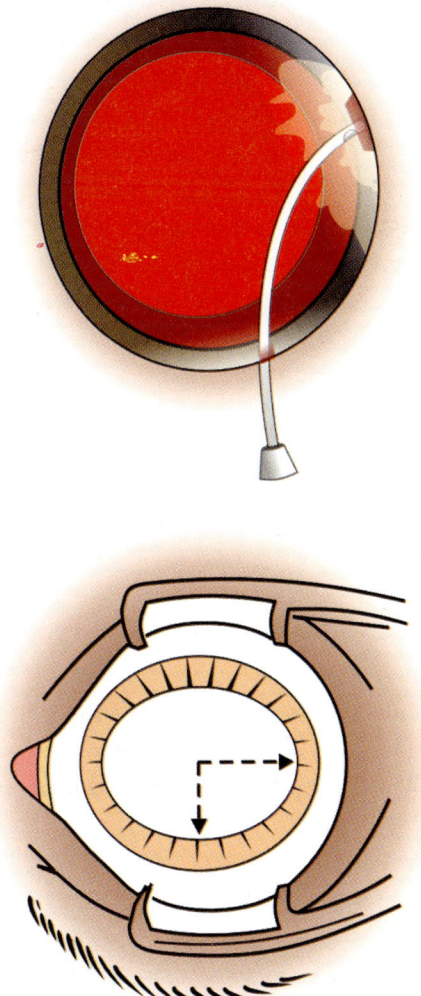

Fig. 4.2: Removal of subincisional cortex with the help of 23 no. cannula from the side port

After doing this step you can revert back and continue doing conventional extracapsular cataract extraction as before.

When the side port incision you have made, is not upto the mark—

Width of incision may be too small and there is leakage of wound. Figure 4.3 showing length, width, depth). Suture it with 10-0 polygalactin and make another incision by the side of previous incision, 1 or 2 mm away.

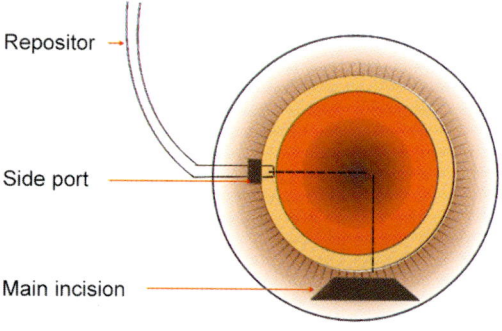

Fig. 4.3: Shows length and width of main incision

Main Phaco Incision: How to Learn?

Please read about theory part in textbooks on phaco. You can learn main phaco incision first on goat's eyeball or eye bank eyes and then on patients. It is affordable to learn with steel keratome initially and then you can shift over to diamond keratome. Size of keratome should be around 2.4 to 3.2 mm. Keratome with a sharp tip should be used, or else there is danger of detachment of Descemet's membrane. This is why steel keratome should be discarded after single use.

While making main incision, fix the eyeball by holding at the margin of side port incision with Huskins forceps or iris repositor (Fig. 4.4) make an incision starting from limbal

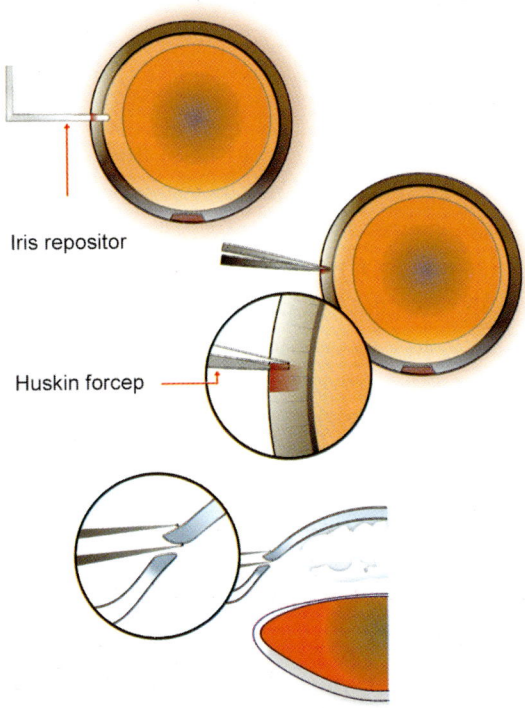

Iris repositor

Huskin forcep

Fig. 4.4: Figure shows how to hold the eyeball with iris repositor and Huskin's forceps

clear cornea. If anterior chamber is very shallow or pupil is constricted, incision should be 1 or 2 mm inside limbus. This of course, will increase the astigmatism, as we are nearer the visual axis. However, the advantage of choosing this site is prevention of iris prolapse and better maneuverability of instruments. There is no need to make any groove. Width of incision should be around 1.5 mm. Depress the cornea slightly so as to create a small dimple, while entering into anterior chamber.

Site of Incision

Once you master the art of incision and phaco, site of incision can be selected as per K- reading. Site of incision should be at steeper meridian, i.e. with a higher diopteric value, for example, if K reading is 42 D at 90 degrees and 45 D at 180 degrees, then steepest meridian is 45 D at 180 degrees and incision will be at 180 degrees. This incision neutralizes the existing astigmatism first.

Do not think of astigmatism when you are learning phaco. It is not the priority item to be mastered. First learn phaco techniques. Then try to reduce astigmatism.

Distance between centers of side port and main incision should be so much that both hands can work together inside anterior chamber comfortably. It should be approximately 7 to 8 mm or the angle between two should be 70 to 90 degrees (Fig. 4.5).

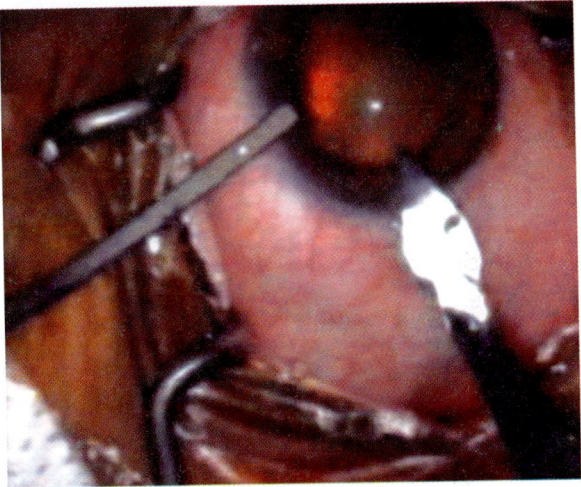

Fig. 4.5: Shows the approximate angle between the side port and main incision, it should be about 70° to 90°

What to do when main phaco incision is not up to the mark?

When the incision size is larger, anterior chamber starts collapsing due to leakage from sides. In this case a temporary 8-0 nylon suture can be placed at the edge of incision to decrease its size and you can continue doing phaco. Otherwise you can close this incision with 10-0 polygalactin and then make new incision shifting your sitting position accordingly.

- In learning phase the incision should be at temporal side only, slightly on right side for right-handed surgeon. Then learn at steepest meridian once the phaco is mastered.

- If Descemet's membrane detachment is noticed and if it is small, you can continue with procedure further. A large detachment however needs to be sutured. After suturing, shift back to extracapsular cataract extraction if you have not yet mastered phaco.

Why corneal incision, why not scleral?

The greatest advantage of temporal clear corneal incision is that you can directly reach nucleus, cracking is easier and rotating nuclear fragments is effort less. In scleral incision, route of entry is zigzag. Therefore, maneuverability of handpiece is difficult and ultimately it becomes difficult to operate or learn phaco. In brief, learning and mastering phaco is easy if you start from clear corneal temporal side (Fig. 4.6). This is one of the very important reasons why in early period surgeons have kept their phaco machines idle, thinking that shifting to phaco was nearly impossible.

Other advantages of temporal clear corneal incisions over routine head end or 12 o'clock incisions are well known.

1. Visual axis being slightly on nasal side, we are away from it. The more you are away from visual axis less astigmatism you create (by same size incision).
2. It can be done under topical anesthesia, as there is no need to take superior rectus suture.

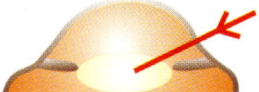

Clear corneal incision: Path of phaco
tip going directly upto the lens nucleus
facilitating maneuverability inside

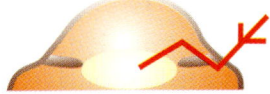

Scleral incision: Zig-zag path traversed
by phaco tip; access to the nucleus
difficult; hampering maneuverability
within

Fig. 4.6: Advantage of clear corneal incision

3. Fluid drains out easily; therefore red glow is better.
   Red glow during surgery is better also because eye
   does not move downwards during surgery.
4. Eighty percent of patients are found to have
   astigmatism against the rule that is steepest meridian is
   at 180 that is neutralised with this incision.

How to avoid corneal hydration near the incision?

Hydration of the corneal wound causes poor visibility.
Although it does not cause any permanent damage to
the tissue, it hampers with clarity of vision while operating. Aim should be to avoid corneal wound hydration. If
the width of corneal incision or tunnel is less, then chances

of getting corneal wound hydrated are less. Another advantage with smaller width is that the maneuvers become easy in the anterior chamber. So a beginner should always try to make the width of tunnel or incision less. However, this creates a problem of increased wound leakage. In spite of all this it is better to have incision with a smaller width and suture it at the end. Once hydration occurs it is almost an irreversible process. After hydration occurs, if you wait for few minutes it may regress slightly. It increases if there is a stretch on wound edges and fluid is coming out. In other words the maneuvers should be such that there is no stretch on edges of wound but it should be used as fulcrum. Secondly, the irrigating holes should not be partly in the wound.

Chapter 5

Phacodynamics

This chapter will stress on salient features, which are of practical importance. I suggest you to read the theory part thoroughly from the textbooks on phaco. I have not included many important aspects on this subject here, which are established beyond doubt and accepted universally. You ought to know them. However, I have mentioned about some vital, practical points on phacodynamics.

Human nature is such that the work, which we do not like, we keep it pending, for example, we are always lazy in reading the theory part. About phacodynamics same thing happens. We think that we will start doing surgery first and then read the theory simultaneously. But this never happens and it neither helps. One has to master the theory of phacodynamics and fluidics thoroughly before to begin with the surgery. Basic aim here is very clear and simple. **Anterior chamber should remain formed throughout the procedure** and at the same time you should not damage the corneal endothelium or posterior capsule. It is like driving on a narrow hilly road where, you have a hill on one side and a valley on the other.

PERISTALTIC PUMP

I am using peristaltic pump phaco machine and I am quite happy with it. The phaco machine pump level should be at eye level. If it is lower or higher, then it may cause problems.

Irrigation

Irrigation is by gravity. Irrigating fluid will stop coming into anterior chamber automatically, if there are no wound leaks and pressure in the anterior chamber equals water column height (usually the irrigating bottle is at 60 to 70 centimeters from patient's eye level). From phaco handpiece, fluid should come out in a stream or jet and not dropwise. This sounds as if some forceful fountain is splashing water. In reality however, when handpiece is inside anterior chamber, fluid does not come with so much force, neither it causes much turbulence. When I started doing Phaco, it used to be my fear that this stream may cause loss of corneal endothelial cells, which, in fact, is not the case. This is because the pressure in anterior chamber is the same as that of pressure in the bottle. Hence, fluid does not come out as a forceful stream inside the anterior chamber. It is just that, whatever amount of fluid comes out of anterior chamber is replaced by irrigating fluid. This is the reason; corneal endothelium is well protected and not damaged by this stream.

It is advisable to **use irrigation tubing of a larger bore** from phaco tip to the irrigation bottle. A TUR set tube used by general surgeons for prostate or abdominal surgeries can suffice the purpose. If the lumen of the tubing is small, it takes longer time to replace the leakage of fluid from anterior chamber. With a large bore, the flow of the fluid is free and fast. Amount of surge (see Surge Phenomenon) becomes less if lumen of the irrigating tube is large. This is very important in reducing surge.

Air entry into the bottle should be free. If airway cannula gets blocked, fluid cannot flow easily. The airway cannula of at least 20-G should be used. The bottle height should be 70 to 90 centimeters from the eye level. Little bit more height of bottle really helps in avoiding surge. Always be watchful, if there is any small kink in the tubing. This will obstruct the easy flow. Kink usually occurs near phaco probe.

Many times if somebody says flow rate in the beginning, novice surgeon may feel it as irrigation flow rate but it is not so. It is aspiration flow rate. Irrigation is by gravity and flow depends on how much fluid is going out of anterior chamber.

Phaco Power

The function of phaco or ultrasonic power is to fragment the nucleus in small pieces. These pieces then get emulsified in the saline and then by vacuum are sucked out. The phaco power varies from zero to 100 percent. By foot-pedal you can increase the power. More you press foot-pedal more you get the power. That means it is linear.

When we make the phaco power on the needle moves to and fro in meridian of the needle, this distance between the movement is termed as 'stroke length'. Now, imagine if initial phaco power is 30 percent and you are increasing it to 60 percent. This means the movement of the phaco tip to and fro (axial stroke length has doubled). It means the span of movement increases but frequency, i.e. cycles per minute will remain same (say about 45000/sec), when you increase the phaco power.

How do you judge that this phaco power is proper for a particular patient (or nucleus)?

After hydrodissection, insert phaco probe. Touch the phaco tip to the nucleus in such a way that nucleus will move by 0.5 or 1 mm in opposite direction. Now press the foot-pedal till there is cutting action of the tip (phaco on), which means that the phaco tip will enter into the substance of nucleus rather than pushing the nucleus ahead. If the nucleus is getting pushed rather than cutting action of tip on the nucleus, it means that phaco power is insufficient and needs to be increased. Keep it little higher than required for sculpting. In fact, it is easy once you are used to the linear progressive action of footswitch (like car accelerator). Even if you set it at higher side, i.e. 60 percent, still you can use only 10 percent or less according to foot-pedal position. As you progressively press the foot-pedal phaco power will progressively increase.

While making a groove in the nucleus, always start from the periphery. Less phaco power is required at periphery, which is a softer area, than in the center of nucleus, which is harder. As you move from periphery to nucleus, go on increasing phaco power and again reduce it by pressure on footswitch as you come from center to periphery. Though appears difficult while reading, this technique can be done smoothly and at ease, once you get tuned to the footswitch. The basic is central core hard nucleus requires more phaco power.

> YOU WILL LEARN MORE ABOUT THE ROAD BY TRAVELLING IT RATHER THAN BY CONSULTING ALL THE MAPS IN THE WORLD!

How to assess the depth of groove that has been created?

If the groove is too deep, it may touch posterior capsule, if it is shallow it becomes difficult to divide nucleus. That's why it needs to be just adequate. Depth can be assessed by several ways.

a. Red glow becomes brighter as compared to other part of nucleus, if you are nearer the posterior capsule.

b. The depth of groove should be so much as to accommodate 3 to 4 phaco tips. To know this, put the phaco tip in the posterior most portion of groove and try to imagine—how many phaco tips it can accommodate. If you feel it can accommodate 3 tips, it means the depth is sufficient and you need not go deeper.

c. It is wiser to learn initially by making a groove and then taking out nucleus by extracapsular cataract extraction. This nucleus should be examined for actual assessment of depth.

SURGE PHENOMENON

Whenever phaco tip is occluded by fragment and the preset vacuum is reached, at this moment if occlusion of phaco tip suddenly gets released (either due to phaco and / or vacuum) the fragment is abruptly pulled into the tip, then the preset vacuum suddenly aspirates or sucks out contents of anterior chamber. This causes sudden collapse of anterior chamber. These happenings are called as **'surge phenomenon'**. Always make it a habit to test the phaco machine for surge phenomenon prior to use every time (Fig. 5.1). During surgery surge should never occur.

How do you test for surge phenomenon?

Set the vacuum and the flow rate to the maximum level that you will be using in that particular patient. Fill the priming chamber with fluid and put it on the phaco hand-piece. Occlude the aspiration tube by kinking the tube manually. This will create an audible signal, indicating that preset vacuum is reached. Now, release the occlusion of aspiration tube. At this time keep the aspiration on and look at the priming chamber. If priming chamber does not collapse it means there is no surge. Consider this as a green signal for starting surgery.

If priming chamber collapses, it means there is surge. The priming chamber mimics the anterior chamber. The priming chamber collapses means anterior chamber will also collapse. This is dangerous as it may cause damage to posterior capsule or endothelium. Now reduce the vacuum and flow rate, till you do not get even slight collapse of priming chamber after repeating the above test. Surgeon should never cross limits of preset vacuum

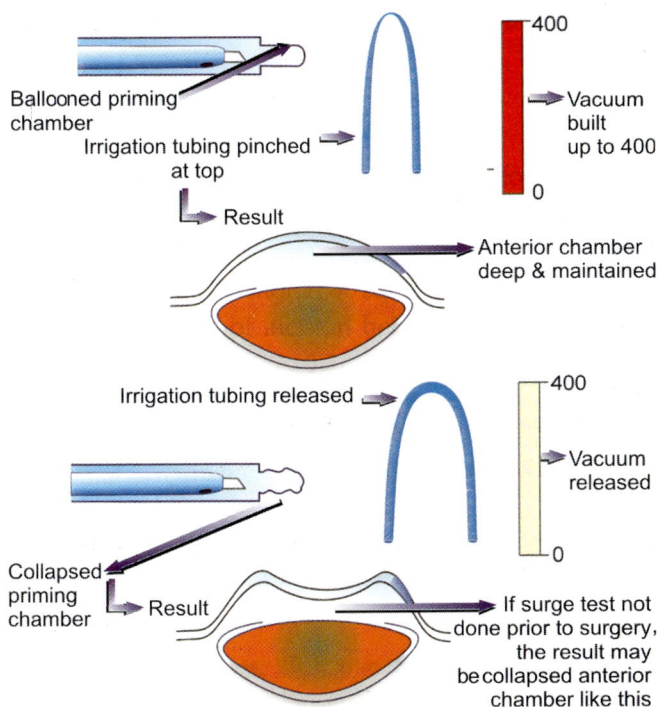

Fig. 5.1: Shows how to test for surge phenomena. If the priming chamber collapses there is surge. Recheck the settings and tubings

and flow rate of that machine to avoid surge while operating. Remember, this test for surge phenomenon should be performed prior to every case.

Causes of Surge

- *Air in the tubing:* This will decrease the fluid entering the anterior chamber. Thus, enough fluid will not be replaced, causing the fluid in anterior chamber to rush in the tubing, causing surge.

- *Fluid coming out from side port:* If the side port is leaking anterior chamber will become shallow. Sometimes the width of the side port or main incision is appropriate but if you press over the lips of the incision, while maneuvering in the chamber then fluid leakage is more and surge develops. So avoid pressing over the lips of the incision. The way to do maneuvers without pressure over the wound edges should be learnt.
- Fluid coming out from main incision.
- *Very small incision:* In case of small incision, the sleeve will get compressed at the incision, decreasing the amount of fluid entering the anterior chamber and may cause surge.
- Kinking of the tubing.

Other Causes

1. No fluid in the bottle
2. Bottle height—if the height is less.
3. Some mechanical problem in the machine (vent not proper).

VACUUM

There are two components of vacuum:
1. Preset vacuum
2. Actual vacuum.

Preset Vacuum

Surgeon can choose and set the preset vacuum.

Imagine that the preset vacuum is set at 300 mm of Hg, which means that at any moment during surgery, vacuum will never go beyond 300 mm of Hg.

The **function of vacuum is to hold** or fix the nucleus or nuclear fragments. This is very essential, as it is difficult to chop a mobile nucleus. More the vacuum, firmer is the grip on nuclear fragment. Naturally, a question strikes our mind, why not to keep vacuum at maximum, i.e. 500 mm of Hg to have a firm grip on fragment? If you do so, when nuclear fragment gets sucked in, sudden surge will be there resulting into collapse of anterior chamber. If this happens, it is real disaster. To avoid this, we keep the actual vacuum, just enough to hold the nucleus firmly. This gives us, a greater safety margin.

How to get a judgment of vacuum needed for any particular nucleus?

Keep the preset vacuum at lower level. Once the phaco tip is embedded or goes inside the nucleus and gets occluded, the preset vacuum is reached. Try to chop. If you feel that the grip on the nucleus is getting released while doing chopping, it means preset vacuum should be increased till you get a firm hold of the nucleus with phaco tip; so that nucleus doesn't get dislodged while chopping. If it does not get dislodged you can try reducing it till it gets dislodged and then increase it little bit so that you get idea of vacuum needed for each type of nucleus. This you can try in goat's eye with introducing the nucleus of routine ECCE. For hard nucleus preset vacuum is more needed than in the soft nucleus. To begin with, you should try on gray nucleus (grade II). Initially, try to get an idea about various types of nuclei and the preset vacuum needed. You can slowly judge this by experience. Naturally, for brittle nucleus it should be less. As you are approaching the fag end of the procedure, i.e. when only one or two nuclear fragments are remaining, vacuum should be reduced. Else, the slight surge will cause posterior capsular touch with phaco probe. When only 1 or 2 fragments are remaining, you do not need to do chopping. You only need to feed these fragments to the handpiece and this requires lesser vacuum.

Actual Vacuum

It means, vacuum present in the tubing at a particular time. This value is never static and will change frequently while operating. This will never be more than preset vacuum level at any moment of time.

When to increase the vacuum

1. The nucleus gets dislodged from the tip when you want to chop. This occurs in spite of tip being completely embedded in nucleus and preset vacuum level being achieved. This is the right time to increase the vacuum.
2. When the chattering is occurring even if the tip is completely occluded and preset vacuum is achieved.

When to decrease the vacuum

If surge phenomenon is there, vacuum needs to be decreased.

What is chattering?

When the nucleus fragment moves to and fro and does not get engaged in the tip with phaco on, this movement is called as chattering.

Chattering can be due to inadequate flow rate or inadequate vacuum. If the tip is completely occluded by the nucleus fragment and then chattering occurs, then this is due to less vacuum. If the tip is not getting completely occluded and then chattering occurs, it means flow rate is less. Sometimes the high phaco power used is also a cause for chattering (See details on page 144).

FLOW RATE

Phaco beginners always presume that flow rate means rate of irrigation. However, it is not so. Flow rate indicates aspiration flow rate in cc/minute and usually ranges from 0 to 40 cc/min.

The main **function of flow rate is to attract (follow ability)** loose fragments of nucleus or cortex towards the probe. When you increase the flow rate, it increases follow ability of these fragments towards probe. Thus, for increasing follow ability, one has to increase flow rate.

Again a question comes to mind, why not set the flow rate at maximum to start with? The reason is, if you keep it at maximum, it will attract posterior capsule as well as iris. This is why we like to keep it at a level just enough to attract loose cortical or nuclear fragments.

If you increase flow rate, and if phaco tip is occluded, preset vacuum is reached faster; this is called as '**Rise**

time'. Rise time, in other words, is time required to reach preset vacuum when the tip is occluded. It will be minimum when the aspiration flow rate is at maximum.

When to increase the flow rate:

1. If nuclear fragment is not getting attracted even if the phaco tip is close to the fragment.
2. If chattering is there and nucleus is not occluding the phaco tip.

- *Before putting phaco machine into use always make it a point to test for Vent Mechanism and Surge Phenomenon prior to every case.*

Testing for Vent Mechanism

For this put priming chamber filled with fluid. Press the footswitch and occlude the aspiration tube. Then allow vacuum to reach preset level. Once this happens, keeping aspiration tube occluded, release the footswitch completely. As soon as footswitch is released, vacuum will come down to zero only if vent mechanism is functioning well. **If this fails to occur, do not use machine till the problem is rectified.** If you use machine then there will be surge.

Testing for Surge Phenomenon

This has been explained already (Refer to Surge Phenomenon).

Chapter 6

Woodcutter's Nucleus Cracking Technique

I always enjoy innovating small little things, new surgical skills and equipment which make my routine work easier, better and enjoyable preventing monotony. In this way I can sail in the ocean of ophthalmology smoothly. Woodcutter's technique of dealing with the nucleus is one such idea born in my mind. I nourished this technique and now I am enjoying its fruits.

Have you anytime watched how a woodcutter cuts a log of wood? When he wants to divide a wooden log, he nails a chisel in the center. Then with an axe he goes on hammering on the wooden log. As he approaches the chisel the wooden log automatically gets divided into two vertical fragments because of the strain created by chisel. (Fig. 6.1). The crack (or cleavage) extends automatically beyond chisel and deep inside too. This creates a vertical crack on both the sides of nail. By this indirect force he can divide the wooden log into two pieces. The procedure that I have named as **'woodcutter's'** technique makes use of a chopper that functions like a chisel stapled in the wooden log and phaco handpiece acts like an axe.

The technique is a boon especially for nuclei that are hard. In this technique we are using phaco tip instead of a chopper to divide nucleus. Chopper only stabilizes nucleus and creates a site of strain that gives direction for crack to develop. The subsequent chapter will tell you more about it.

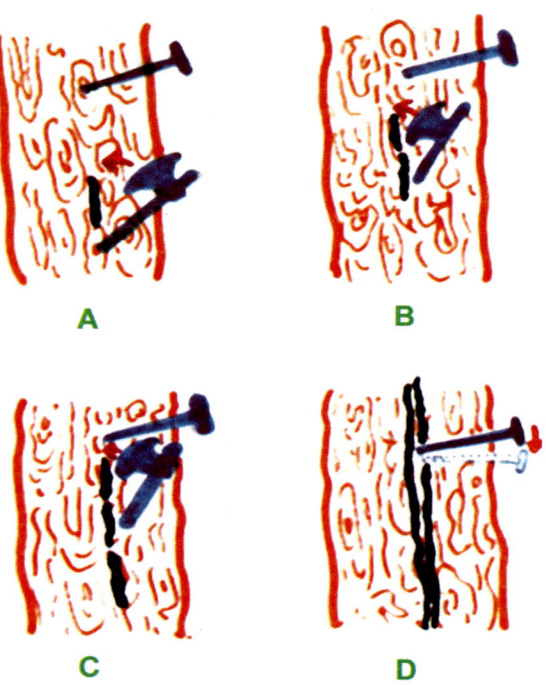

Figs 6.1A to D: A. Shows how the chisel has been hammered at one point. **B.** Shows how the axe hammers. **C.** Shows how the axe hammers upto the chisel. But not beyond it. **D.** Shows how the crack has been extended beyond the chisel

ITS NOT ONLY MACHINERY THAT BECOMES OBSOLETE; OBSOLESCENCE OF MIND ALSO STOPS YOUR GROWTH SO, TRY BEING INNOVATIVE.

How Woodcutter's technique differs from the chop technique?

The woodcutter technique involves **cracking** technique, whereas the chop technique involves cutting. If you want to divide any firm object using a sharp instrument, it is easy to cut it. However, this cut will resemble a stab wound. The cut will not extend beyond the portion of entry of the sharp instrument within that object. It will be limited only to that portion through which the sharp instrument, has traveled (Figs 6.1 E and F). As against this, when we use cracking (woodcutter's) technique, the cleavage extends deeper and much beyond the passage of the cracking instrument i.e. towards periphery, although the instrument does not touch this portion. Same thing happens while cutting a wooden log. The woodcutter will never hammer beyond the chisel (Fig. 6.2). In spite of this crack develops beyond the insertion point of the chisel. Similarly the stroke of his hammer never involves the entire

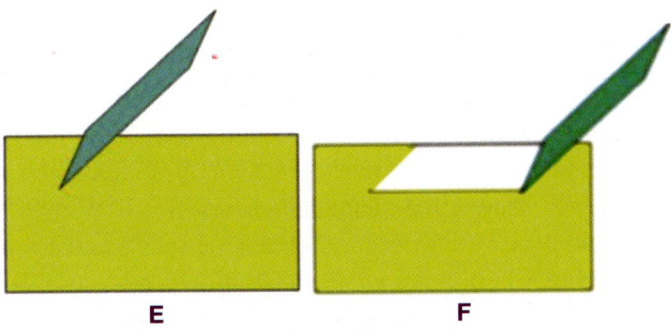

E	**F**

Figs 6.1E and F: Cutting techniques

CHOP TECHNIQUE

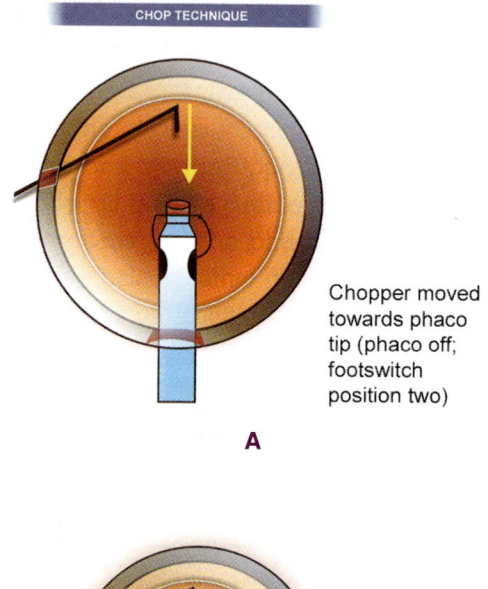

Chopper moved towards phaco tip (phaco off; footswitch position two)

A

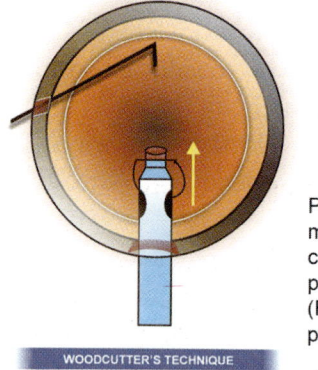

Phaco tip moving towards chopper with phaco on (Footswitch position three)

WOODCUTTER'S TECHNIQUE

B

Figs 6.2A and B: Nucleus cracking
A. Chop technique. **B.** Woodcutter's technique

depth of the log but still the crack involves entire depth. Woodcutter's technique works on same principle. We get a crack in the nucleus that extends till periphery and also deep inside the posterior part of nucleus. This happens in spite of the fact that the chopper and phaco tip never go beyond half thickness of the nucleus.

Similarly, if you take a wooden strip and embed four nails involving only half thickness of this, the result will be a crack that extends beyond the embedded nails involving entire depth. This happens even if you have not touched the part of strip beyond nails and the nails have not entered full thickness, and still you get the crack involving full thickness (Fig. 6.3).

To stress more on cracking technique I shall like to quote another example. If you hammer a chisel on a stone, the moment chisel enters some depth, a crack develops and the stone automatically cracks into several pieces. Thus, the chisel has not entered the entire depth of stone and still crack involves entire depth.

In brief, ***chopping technique is a cutting technique; whereas woodcutter's technique is a cracking technique.*** In chopping technique you have to tear the attachments of nuclear fragments while in woodcutter's technique crack is already till the posterior capsule. Only thing you need to do is to go certain depth (30 to 40%) just separate the two pieces.

What is the role of thickness of nucleus?

In extracapsular and small incision cataract surgery there is no role of thickness of the nucleus. But in phaco surgery

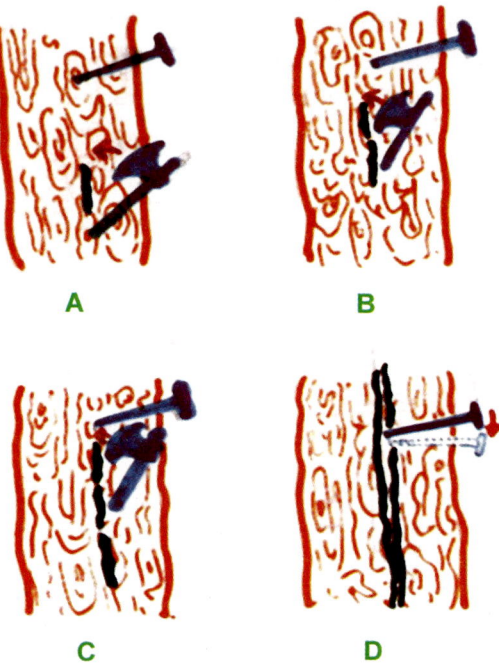

Figs 6.3A to D: A. Shows how the chisel has been hammered at one point. **B.** Shows how the axe hammers. **C.** Shows how the axe hammers upto the chisel. But not beyond it. **D.** Shows how the crack has been extended beyond the chisel

there is a definite role of thickness of nucleus, especially in woodcutter's nucleus cracking or chop technique. In woodcutters' nucleus cracking technique, it is necessary that your phaco tip should go deep into nucleus and the chopper should go about 30 to 40 percent deep. Thus, estimating the thickness of nucleus pays an important role in woodcutters' technique. If your phaco tip or chopper does not achieve the adequate depth, you cannot get the full thickness crack. You may get a groove instead of crack if you have not gone 40 percent deep.

If the nucleus is thick, as in hard sclerotic cataracts the following changes are made:

- Exposed part of the phaco tip should be kept more, about 2.0 mm
- More power is required to embed the nucleus
- Higher vacuum is required to hold the nucleus
- Flow rate should be more
- Chopper should go deep
- Phaco tip should go deep.

How to assess the thickness of nucleus?

In initial stages, when you may have to convert from phaco to ECCE because of one or the other reason. This is the right time to assess the thickness of the nucleus. Suppose you have made a groove and because some reason you have converted to ECCE. When you deliver the nucleus see the depth of groove you have made. Here you come to know that you should have gone still deeper. As well as you know how thick is this particular nucleus. Thus, each time you convert see for the depth you have reached. Gradually you learn to assess for the thickness of a particular nucleus.

DEALING WITH NUCLEUS AND ITS FRAGMENTS USING WOODCUTTER'S NUCLEUS CRACKING TECHNIQUE

This woodcutter's nucleus cracking technique is the

excellent way to deal with harder nuclei like grade II, III, and IV.

Important Pre-requisite

Phaco sleeve should be 1.5 to 2 mm behind the outermost point of phaco needle. The exposed part of tip (portion of the phaco needle, which is not covered by sleeve) should be slightly more as compared to that required for routine chop technique (Fig. 6.4). If you keep part of tip exposed very small, then phaco tip entering inside the nucleus is small and instead of division you get a groove in nucleus. For a harder nucleus tip exposed should be more. If part of tip exposed is more than required, the disadvantage is that irrigation may stop even if you

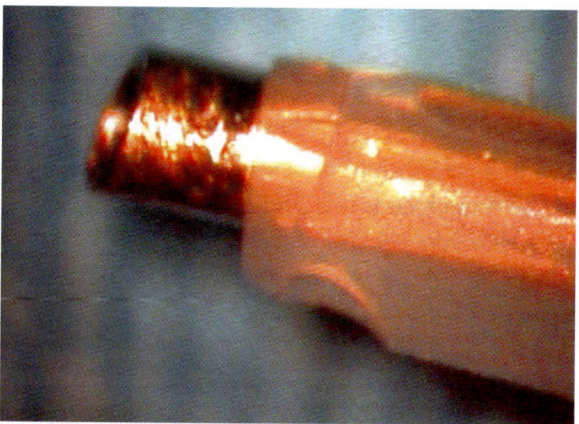

Fig. 6.4: Shows exposed part of phaco tip. It is usually kept more in woodcutter's technique

withdraw phaco hand piece slightly. (This is because the irrigation ports come near the incision and get covered by incision).

For this technique there is no need of sculpting. Similarly no need to make a groove in nucleus. This technique can be directly applied to divide nucleus.

Steps of Woodcutter's Technique

1 Part of the phaco needle, which is not covered by sleeve, should be slightly more as discussed earlier.
2. The instruments, i.e. phaco-needle and chopper are introduced inside in the anterior chamber.
3. Push the nucleus slightly (by one millimeter) to opposite clock position (opposite to the incision site) with the help of a chopper (Fig. 6.5).
4. Embed the phaco tip into the nucleus. **You should enter keeping handpiece 70 to 80 degrees vertical** (Fig. 6.6). The advantage of this is that the tip gets fully embedded inside before you reach the

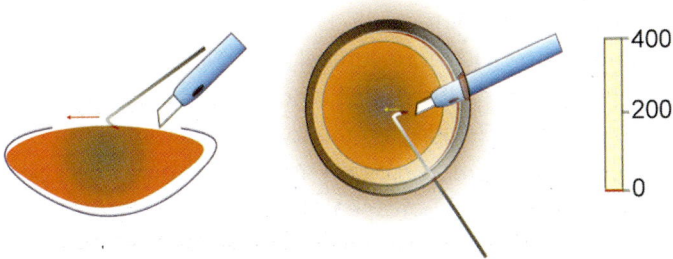

Fig. 6.5: Shows how the chopper pushes the nucleus towards opposite side, i.e. about 1 mm

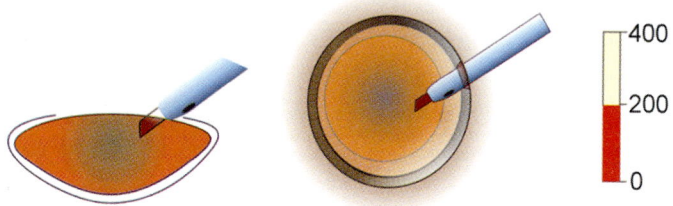

Fig. 6.6: Shows the position of phaco probe. It should be more vertical, about 70 to 80 degree

center of nucleus or center of capsulorhexis. The phaco tip should get embedded 30 to 40 percent thickness of nucleus.

5. When the preset vacuum is reached, move the nucleus towards incision site by one mm (Fig. 6.7). Embed the chopper at capsulorhexis margin into the nucleus. The chopper should reach 30 to 40 percent depth of nucleus. This is possible only when you are holding the nucleus firmly with phaco tip. Many times novice surgeon feels that the sharp tip of chopper may cause rent in posterior capsule. But this is not possible if the chopper is held more vertical as shown in Figure 6.8A. The chopper is held as if whole nucleus is pushed in the phaco tip. This way the force of vacuum and your chopper action force are in similar direction. See chapter Action That Speaks For Them.

6. Push the phaco tip **with phaco on** towards the chopper (Fig. 6.8B). This will break the nucleus into two vertical fragments in nearly all the cases (Fig. 6.9). If not, then

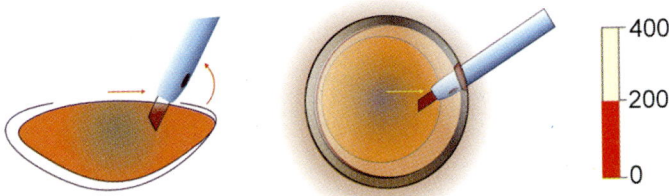

Fig. 6.7: Shows how the nucleus is pulled towards incision after embeding the probe into the nucleus. The point to be noted here is that you should use the incision as a fulcrum

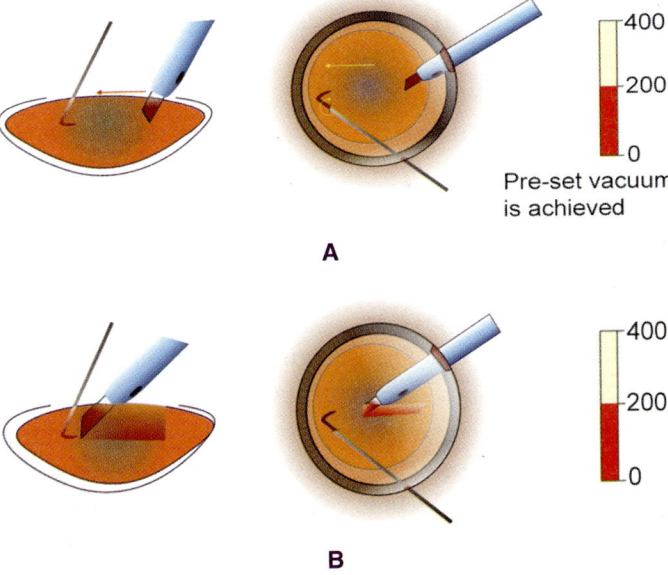

Pre-set vacuum is achieved

A

B

Figs 6.8A and B: A. Shows how the position of the chopper is vertical. As if whole nucleus is pushed in phaco tip. **B.** Shows the correct position of chopper (vertical) and phaco probe. Push the phaco probe with phaco on towards the chopper

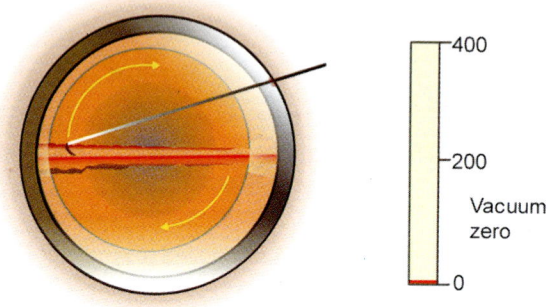

Fig. 6.9: Shows how full thickness crack
has been developed

introduce the chopper into the depth of the crack that
you have made and try to separate two fragments
from each other. It is necessary to go to the base of
the crack with chopper because it is easier to displace
fragments without stretch on zonules. If still you cannot
divide the nucleus, which may happen in the beginning
then rotate the nucleus by 180 degrees. If rotation is
not possible, repeat hydrodissection. Try to rotate again.
Once rotation is complete through 180 degree, again
perform the same procedure as mentioned earlier.

7. For second crack (Fig. 6.10) or cleavage rotate the
   nucleus. The previous groove (which is created by
   movement of phaco tip towards the chopper) gives
   you space. (You get more space as hard central part is
   taken out). This space can be utilized for inserting
   phaco needle in the center and again dividing the
   nucleus in above-mentioned manner.

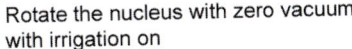

Rotate the nucleus with zero vacuum
with irrigation on

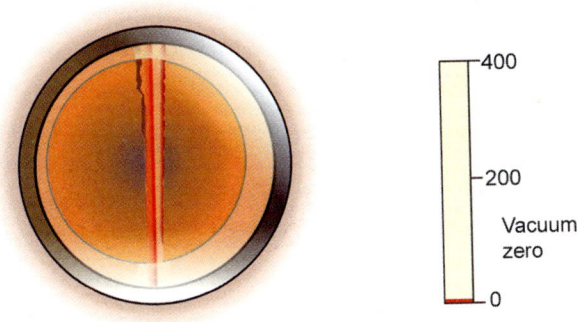

Embed the phaco tip directly in the centre of thickness
of nucleus and make a second crack after pre-set vacuum
is achieved

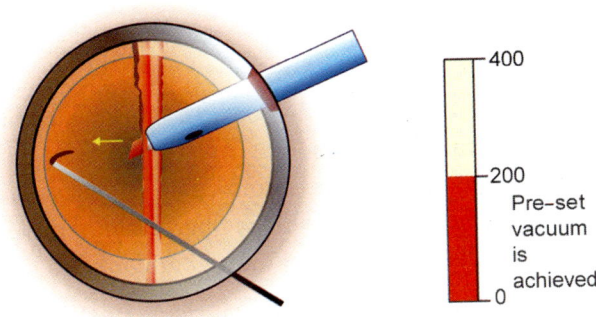

Fig. 6.10: Showing how the nucleus is rotated after first crack,
keeping vacuum zero. For second crack you get a space in
center and then second crack is done

8. The procedure is repeated till small fragments of nucleus are made (Fig. 6.11).

   In most of the cases you will be able to achieve fragmentation of nucleus into two pieces; except in very soft nuclei.

> ## THE HARD STUFF IS EASY;
> ## THE SOFT STUFF IS HARD.

9. *Continuous irrigation:* In initial stages one can make use of continuous irrigation mode in the phaco machine. The advantage of this mode is that you do not have to go to irrigation mode every time. You have to concentrate on position 2 and 3 only. Learning foot- switch operation becomes easy as there are only two steps.

Advantages of Woodcutter's Technique

Woodcutter technique is basically a cracking technique and not a cutting technique.

   While making division of nucleus you are always away from posterior capsule. Hence there is no danger of rupturing it. Let us see what are the advantages.

1. The chopper stabilizes the nucleus. Because of this, stretch on zonules is less. This is why I am using phaco power to divide nucleus rather than chopper. Chopper only stabilizes nucleus, and gives direction for crack to develop. As told earlier, chopper can be

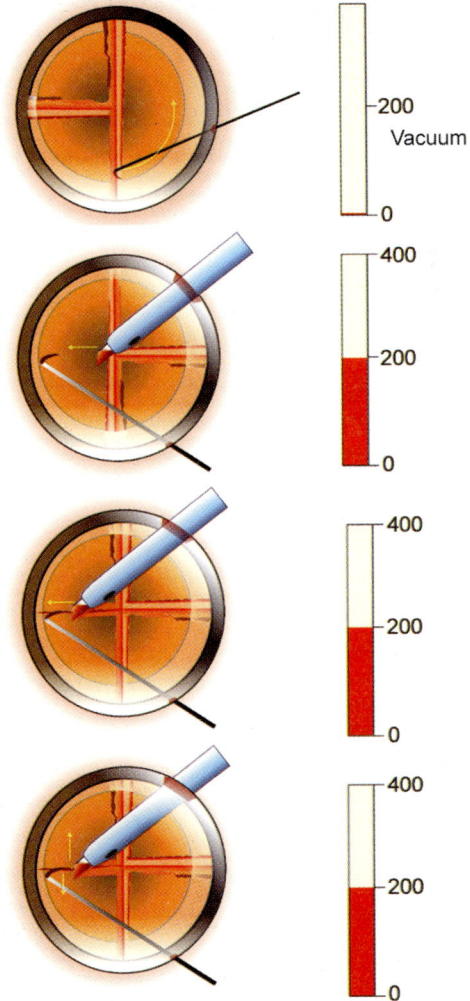

Fig. 6.11: Shows how four quadrant cracking is done

compared to the chisel stapled in the log of wood and phaco to the axe.

2. As you are in the nucleus and then using phaco power, even if power is more, it will not get dissipated towards, corneal endothelium, which minimizes endothelial damage.

3. You get more space in the center as hard part is taken out when we move the phaco tip towards the chopper with phaco on.

4. You can increase vacuum to a great extent. Even if there is a slight surge, it won't cause many harms as posterior capsule is far away and there is nucleus in between phaco tip and posterior capsule.

5. Less power is required as phaco is done after stabilizing nucleus with chopper as if you are feeding the nucleus in the phaco tip.

6. Division is in one stroke most of times especially in hard nucleus.

7. Less phaco time is required as division is in one stroke. The procedure is fast to perform. Secondly, hard part of nucleus is taken out easily as if you feed it to the needle while moving phaco needle towards chopper.

8. Cleavage extends beyond and deep in the substance of nucleus because of strain created by chopper.

9. We may feel that phaco needle will touch the chopper. But this will not happen because nucleus gets fragmented into two, even before you reach up to the chopper. That's why you will never go up to

equator, i.e. peripheral soft part of nucleus. The needle can become hot as phaco is on with tip occluded.

10. In small pupil or small capsulorhexis it is possible to divide the nucleus as you do not have to go to the periphery and still you get the division of nucleus.

AREAS OF ADDITIONAL ATTENTION (AAA)

Woodcutter's technique, I think is very simple procedure and easier even for phaco beginners. It is easy to master it with clear corneal incision as compared with scleral, because approach is direct in clear corneal incision and manipulations are easy. The needle can become hot as phaco is on with tip occluded.

We may feel that phaco needle will touch the chopper. But this will not because nucleus gets fragmented into two, even before you reach up to the chopper. That's why you will never go up to equator, i.e. peripheral soft part of nucleus.

What do you do when you feel that woodcutter's technique is not working up to the mark?

WE MUST ACCEPT FINITE DISAPPOINTMENT. BUT WE MUST NEVER LOOSE INFINITE HOPES.

1. Please note that woodcutter's technique will not work in very soft nuclei. In this case other procedures are easier and it is not necessary to go for woodcutters.

2. If the sleeve of phaco needle is not pulled back so as to get 1.25 to 1.5 mm of bare area, and then phaco tip will not be able to penetrate in the depth of nucleus, which should be approximately 30 to 40 percent.

3. For grade IV, hard nuclei, distance between phaco tip and sleeve should be more—around 1.5 to 1.75 mm. Here, you should not be afraid that you might go deeper and rupture posterior capsule. This doesn't happen, because hard nuclei are more than 4 mm in thickness antero-posteriorly. Sleeve will not allow tip to go beyond 1.75 mm. So you always have a safety zone of 2 mm around hard nucleus.

4. It is better to learn with clear corneal incision.

5. The angle of phaco handpiece should be more vertical (70 or 80 degrees) (Fig. 6.12). There should be good hold of nucleus before the tip reaches the center of capsulorhexis. Then only you get enough space to move the tip towards chopper and get division of nucleus. If you get hold of nucleus when the tip reaches periphery then it is difficult to perform this procedure, as there is no space to move the phaco tip towards chopper with phaco on.

6. While embedding the tip in the nucleus, in order to have good hold, beginner may keep phaco continuously on even after the sleeve touches the nucleus. This results in loosening the grip. This is because the tip cannot go deeper, but vibrations of the tip enlarge the hole created by the entry of the tip. Thus, the grip by pressure of surrounding nucleus is lost. So stop phaco power utilization immediately

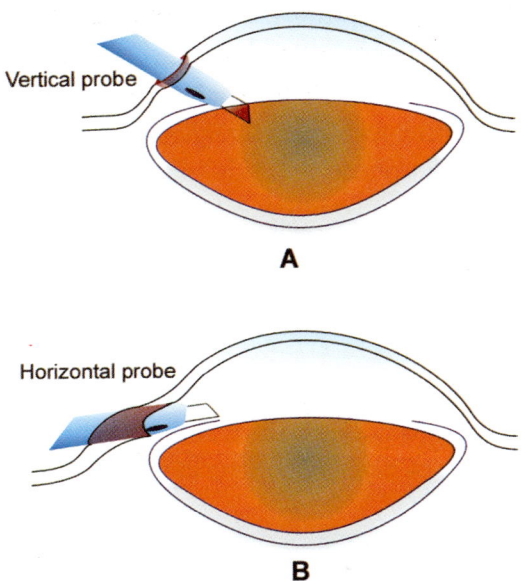

Fig. 6.12: Shows how the probe is held vertical (A) i.e.
70° to 80° and not horizontal (B)

when sleeve touches the nucleus. Usually sleeve
touches the nucleus first on posterior side. This has to
be observed.

How to learn?

LESSONS ARE NOT GIVEN
THEY ARE ALWAYS TAKEN.

For a Phaco Beginner

After you have mastered sculpting and making partial
thickness groove you can directly start learning

woodcutter's technique. This can be better learnt by replacing nucleus in goat's eye by nucleus from stored eye bank eyes, which are not useful for keratoplasty. By this you get exact feeling of having operated on patient's eye. Make main phaco and side port incision on goat's eye. Then do capsulorhexis. Make a larger self-sealing incision of about 6 mm on goat's eye from opposite side. Then push the nucleus taken out from the eye bank eye through the large incision. Embed this nucleus in soft cortex of goat's eye by passing through capsulorhexis. Then suture the large incision. Now learn woodcutter technique on this nucleus. For that matter you can learn any technique of dividing nucleus in this way.

For Phaco Master

Follow the steps (see above) in grade three or four cataract. Do not get disheartened even if you are unable to do it in first case. The technique shall not do any harm to the patient's eye even if it fails. Gradually you shall be master enjoying the fruits of learning this technique.

How to deal with small nucleus fragments at periphery? (Fig. 6.13)

If a small fragment of nucleus remains in the periphery, hold the phaco tip near it and press the footswitch till aspiration is on. The nucleus gets attracted towards the phaco tip. If this does not happen, then we can press the footswitch more so as to activate the phaco power for fraction of seconds. This attracts the nucleus piece toward

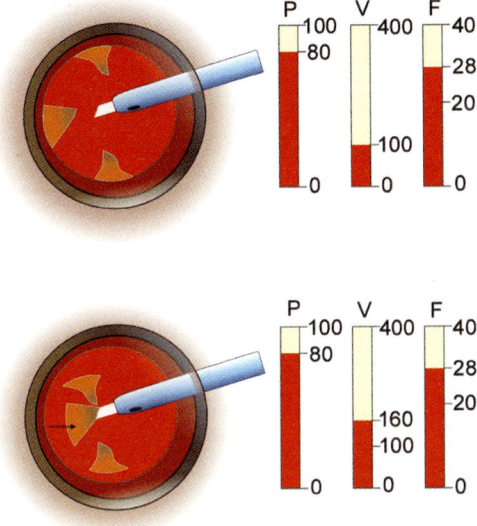

Fig. 6.13: Shows how the handpiece is moved towards the fragments and then aspiration is made. This will attract the fragment to the center. Now you can aspirate the fragment with phaco on

the phaco tip. This is because the tip may be partially blocked by the fine nucleus material. This is more common for micro phaco tips. When we activate the phaco for fraction of seconds, the block gets cleared and nucleus fragment automatically gets attracted towards the phaco tip. Secondly, by making phaco power on for fraction of seconds some turbulence is created that loosens the fragment and attracts it towards the tip.

Chapter 7

Dealing with Epinucleus and Cortex

After taking out the nucleus, especially when hydro-delineation is not done, soft cortical matter is the only thing that we have to remove. If hydrodelineation is done, then epinucleus, which is slightly harder than cortex, remains to be removed.

How to learn?

Cortical matter can be removed using Simcoe cannula with which all of us are well versed in routine extracapsular cataract extraction. Gradually, you can shift over to automated irrigation aspiration. Remember, for this the incision size should be around 2.8 mm and there should not be wound leakage from main or side port incision. Keep the vacuum around 300 and flow rate around 30 (just below maximum level). Deepen the anterior chamber with hydroxypropyl methylcellulose. Then introduce the irrigation aspiration probe. Injecting hydroxypropyl methylcellulose prior to irrigation aspiration helps a lot. It does not allow the posterior capsule to get caught easily. First try to aspirate out cortical matter that is lying at opposite clock position of incision site. This procedure should be practiced at least in 10 cases so that you get an idea about fluidics and dynamics of irrigation and aspiration. Remaining cortical matter can be aspirated by Simcoe cannula. The sub-incisional cortex can be aspirated through side port incision by **dry aspiration technique** or by bimanual technique (Fig. 7.1, see page 115).

Once you master the technique of removing cortical matter from all the sites except sub-incisional cortex (for

Subincisinal cortex removal

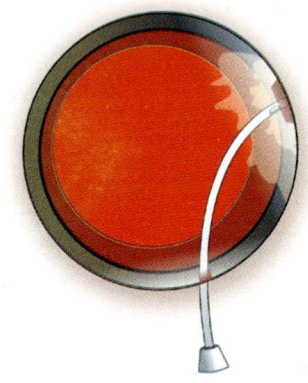

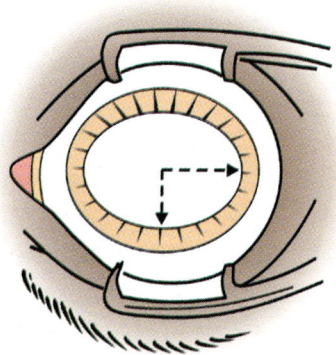

Fig. 7.1: Shows how the dry aspiration is
done with 23 no cannula

which you will use dry aspiration technique), its time to
learn how to remove sub-incisional cortex with automated
irrigation aspiration.

Steps while shifting over to automated irrigation aspiration—Ideal Procedure:

- Keep the vacuum and flow rate at maximum.
- Assure that there is no wound leakage from either of the incisions. It will be a closed chamber irrigation and aspiration.
- Anterior chamber should be maintained throughout procedure. If anterior chamber is getting collapsed, assess what is the reason behind it and rectify all the pitfalls and shortcomings (Page 75, chapter 5).
- While aspirating out the cortical contents try to take out cortex in single large piece or large chunks rather than piece meal. It is very difficult to aspirate out very small fragments of less than 0.3 mm with automated irrigation and aspiration.
- Just bring phaco handpiece near the cortical matter. The cortical matter gets attracted towards port because of existing vacuum and high flow rate. Once it gets attracted then move your handpiece to the site where large chunk of cortical matter is adherent. Move the tip side ways so that central anterior part of full chunk is inside the tip. Never go up to equator. Once the central part of anterior cortex is in the tip now pull it towards the center. Be inside the capsulorhexis margin slightly. If epinucleus or cortical matter is blocking the aspiration port thereby shooting vacuum up to its maximum, using Sinski hook or a lens dialer with other hand try to feed the cortex. This can enhance aspiration. But if it gets sucked out on it's own it is

better as there is no leak from side-port. If we keep the dialer in the side-port constantly then leak of fluid is there. If you want to enhance the aspiration then move the tip in central part in circular fashion this enhances the aspiration.

How to remove sub-incisional cortex?

Anterior chamber should be deep while doing this procedure. If you encounter difficulty, push some hydroxypropyl methylcellulose in the anterior chamber to deepen it. Introduce a 23 gauge cortex aspiration cannula, through side port. The opening of this cannula is facing the cornea and a 2 ml hydroxypropyl methylcellulose syringe attached to it. Now try to aspirate subincisional cortex from side port incision. Whenever you want to remove cannula, push some hydroxypropyl methylcellulose inside. Never move the cannula when you are aspirating. The advantage of this is that even if you catch anterior or posterior capsule, you will not rupture it. If you move the cannula while aspirating, there is a danger of producing a rent. If you happen to see posterior capsule getting pulled inside the port, don't panic. Just push some hydroxypropyl methylcellulose and capsule will be out of port. This is the reason I will again warn you against moving cannula. Whenever you want to move cannula, pushing hydroxypropyl methylcellulose always is a good habit.

TAKE TIME TO THINK, IT HELPS . . .
DON'T JUST REACT!

Removal of subincisional cortex is easy through side port incision, if this incision is 1 to 1.5 mm inside the limbus. Maneuverability of cannula is easy if side port incision is towards center or away from limbus.

Other methods of removing subincisional cortex are with automated irrigation aspiration handpiece and bimanual (Fig. 7.2).

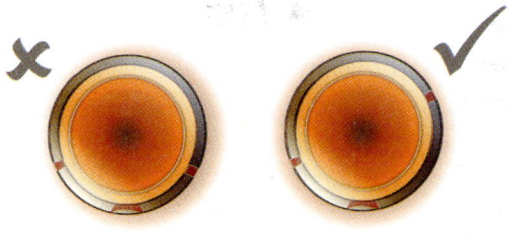

Fig. 7.2: Shows how side ports are made for bimanual irrigation aspiration

When automated irrigation aspiration is needed. The opening of the automated irrigation aspiration port should be at the level of capsulorhexis border so the cortex is pealed out. You are away from the posterior capsule; there is less danger of capture of posterior capsule.

If some cortical matter remains at periphery but is not visible due to constricted pupil, then hold the irrigation aspiration probe near the cortical matter going beneath the iris and make aspiration on. This usually aspirates the cortical matter. Because of flow rate the loose fragments are attracted and aspirated. This procedure is rather blind and may not be visible to you. However, do not move the aspirating tip as it may catch the posterior capsule or anterior capsule which might lead to a rent or zonular dehiscence. You need to make vent on by releasing the footswitch before making irrigation on or moving the aspiration tip.

In an undilated pupil (see page 205 and 206 also) when you are not sure whether aspiration of cortex is complete or not, take out the aspiration handpiece first and then push hydroxypropyl methylcellulose. This results in slight dilatation of the pupil. Look for other sites if any cortical matter is remaining. If so then I use iris hook to retract the iris. Then with posterior capsule polisher like Nightingale ring polisher I loosen the cortical matter from its attachment. Once this is done I insert irrigation-aspiration tip to aspirate the cortical matter as explained above. Let me stress again on the fact that if I want to move the tip I shall move only after bringing footswitch to zero (i.e. vent on position). So even if you have capsule in the tip it will get released. After this you can move the handpiece towards center and remove the remnants. Moving the aspirating tip below the iris, we may land up in dreaded complication like capture of posterior or anterior capsule. But if we avoid moving the tip of irrigation aspiration handpiece and instead make vent on (or bring footswitch position to zero) then even if we catch the capsule it will not cause any problem, as it will be automatically released by vent on.

How do you identify that posterior capsule is caught in the aspiration port? What is the remedy?

If the posterior capsule gets sucked in the aspiration port you will notice **star folds against the red glow** background. Whenever you suspect that posterior capsule is getting pulled, our natural reflex works in such a way that we try to withdraw the handpiece immediately. This leads to another disaster of bringing posterior capsule out. Here is a moment when you have to put yourself into action of not doing anything. Just cool down; release the footswitch. Never move your hand, but foot. Never remove your hand till you release posterior capsule.

LET US LEARN TO SEE A DOOR WHERE OTHERS SEE A WALL

Bimanual Irrigation/Aspiration

The biggest advantage of bimanual is that aspiration port can have easy access at any clock position of capsular bag. So the cortex lying at any place can be easily aspirated. The basis of automated irrigation and aspiration is that it will work only if large chunks of cortex are present. For small fragments it is better to do bimanual. As in automated irrigation aspiration, the aspiration port size is more than 0.3 mm and unless and until the aspiration port gets occluded the vacuum is not build up. So thready cortical matter can not be easily aspirated by automated irrigation aspiration. While for aspiration of small threadlike cortical matter the bimanual is better as the aspiration port size is less than 0.3.

For doing bimanual, make an incision with 20 gauge needle (Fig. 7.3). Or, with MVR blade, make another side port at a site, nearly opposite to the previous side-port. You can use cortex aspiration cannula attached to the aspiration line of phaco machine and irrigation cannula to the irrigation line. Inject hydroxypropyl methylcellulose and deepen the chamber. Push irrigation cannula and make irrigation on and now insert the aspiration cannula. Once both are inside then only start aspiration. Throughout the procedure anterior chamber should not collapse. If it is collapsing then stop aspiration and reduce the preset vacuum. You can exchange the sites of entry of aspiration and irrigation port. So that cortical matter at any clock position can be aspirated (Fig. 7.3). The side ports made for bimanual irrigation aspiration should be diagonally

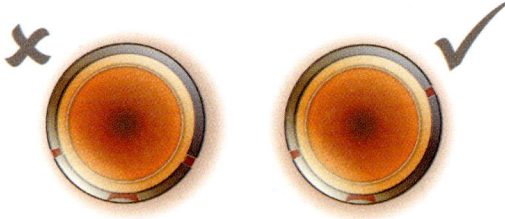

Fig. 7.3: Shows how the side ports are made for bimanual irrigation aspiration. The two side ports should be diagonally opposite to each other, so that it becomes easier to aspirate the cortex at any site including subincisional

opposite to each other and not near to each other, as shown in Figure 7.3. If they are near to each other then again you will feel difficulty in aspirating the subincisional cortex. If they are diagonally opposite it becomes easier to aspirate the cortex at any site including the subincisional cortex.

Capsule polishing can be done by irrigation aspiration handpiece by keeping very low vacuum. You need very low vacuum as irrigating fluid coming in with closed chamber will go out through the aspiration port automatically and that will take the small cortical fibers along with it. I along with this use Knitangle ring polisher. This helps in dislodging the fibers, which are at equator. This is especially useful when the pupil is not fully dilated and visibility of the equatorial lens fibers is not there.

Variation of Bimanual Irrigation Aspiration

Sometimes AC maintainer cannula also can be used in doing bimanual irrigation/aspiration. The cannula of AC maintainer is inserted into one side port and the cortex is aspirated from other side port, which is diagonally opposite. The advantage of this AC maintainer is that it keeps the anterior chamber deep as the irrigation port is large size as compared to routine bimanual irrigation. Thus, it makes easier to aspirate the cortex, as well as the chances of posterior capsular rent decrease to great extent. The other advantage of this is surgeon gets free hand to aspirate with syringe attached to 23 gauge cortex aspiration cannula.

Chapter 8

Frequently Asked Questions

ITS NOT THAT WE CAN NOT SEE
THE SOLUTION
ITS THAT WE SHOULD SEE
THE PROBLEM

Anterior Chamber getting shallower, while operating...

This is a danger signal. If this happens, take out the handpiece (Flow Chart 8.1) See for options A and B –

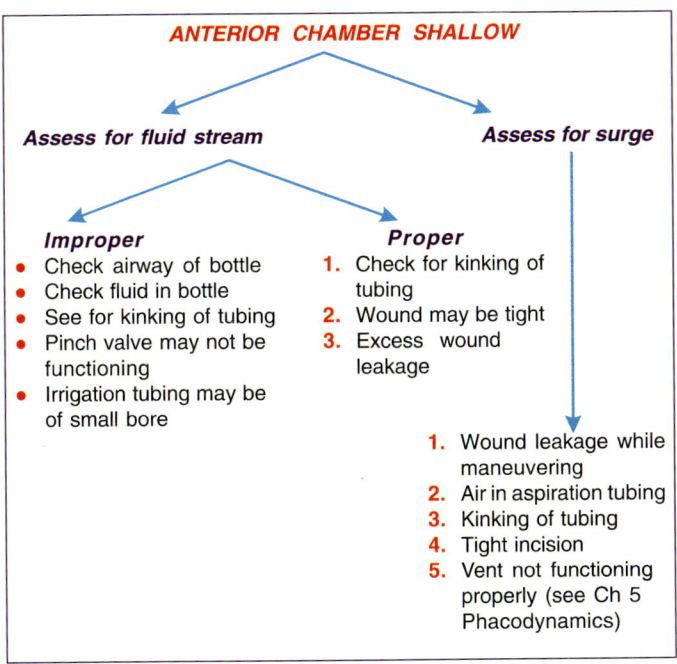

ANTERIOR CHAMBER SHALLOW

Assess for fluid stream

Assess for surge

Improper
- Check airway of bottle
- Check fluid in bottle
- See for kinking of tubing
- Pinch valve may not be functioning
- Irrigation tubing may be of small bore

Proper
1. Check for kinking of tubing
2. Wound may be tight
3. Excess wound leakage

1. Wound leakage while maneuvering
2. Air in aspiration tubing
3. Kinking of tubing
4. Tight incision
5. Vent not functioning properly (see Ch 5 Phacodynamics)

Flow Chart 8.1: What to do when anterior chamber collapses

A. Assess for fluid stream—take out the handpiece and see fluid stream coming from phaco handpiece handle—this may be improper or proper.

Improper

Fluid should come in two separate streams. If this is not the case it means, flow from phaco handpiece is inadequate. See if—

a. Airway of bottle is proper.
b. Fluid in bottle is very less or exhausted.
c. There is kinking of tube near phaco handpiece (See Fig. 8.1).
d. Pinch valve of machine is not functioning properly.
e. Irrigation tubing may be of small bore.

Proper

If fluid stream coming out from handpiece is proper, problem may be:

a. Kinking of irrigation tube. This occurs only when the phaco handpiece is inserted in anterior chamber. This usually occurs near the handpiece (Fig. 8.1).
b. Tight wound compressing the phaco sleeve.
c. Wound leakage: watch for fluid coming out from phaco incision or side port.

   If wound leakage is excessive, you need to suture that incision. Slight hydration of wound may reduce the wound leakage from side port. Sometimes small fragments of nucleus or cortex occluding the incision site may help in reducing wound leakage.

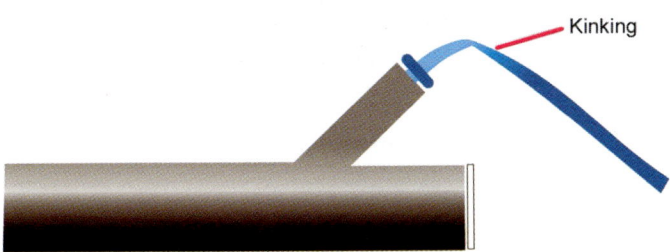

Fig. 8.1: Shows how the kinking of the tube occurs near the phaco handpiece. And how it is avoided with another tube

B. Assess for Surge Phenomenon

Take some fluid in priming chamber and test for surge phenomenon (see page 75, chapter 5). If surge is positive, then reduce vacuum and flow rate till there is no demonstrable surge in priming chamber. Throughout procedure you will never increase vacuum and flow rate beyond this stipulated level.

What are the things, that are suspicious for rent in posterior capsule or zonulolysis?

Cases, which are prone for zonulolysis, are cases with pseudo-exfoliation, hypermature-shrunken cataract, traumatic cataract, subluxated lens, congenital weakness of posterior capsule as in posterior polar cataract and Phacodonesis. Phacodonesis is movement of lens when you introduce handpiece and start irrigation or when you take out the probe. In all such cases where you anticipate weak zonules, some precautions are to be taken, for example, incision site should be away from weak zonule site, preferably at opposite clock position. While doing capsulorhexis anterior chamber depth should be maintained. Too deep anterior chamber also creates problems. As this displaces the subluxated lens posteriorly. There should be least strain on zonules, which are weak (For details see page 201). There should be minimal strain on zonules while manipulating. Once rhexis is complete endocapsular ring (ECR) is inserted. While inserting ECR with dialer from side port, you should give direction to the ring and with suture tying forceps ring is inserted through phaco incision. Phaco procedure in these cases should be done with lesser vacuum and lesser flow rate than normal. There are more chances of posterior capsule getting attracted towards phaco handpiece because it is a mobile structure. This is why we have to be cautious and keep vacuum and flow rate below normal. All manipulations like chopping will be towards area of weak zonules so that there is less stretch on weak zonules. ECR remains permanently in the bag and IOL is put in usual manner. The loops should be right angled to the weak zonular area. Whenever you encounter problem at any step, you can convert to routine extracapsular cataract extraction and if not possible then intracapsular cataract extraction procedure.

Signs of Rent

Anterior chamber suddenly deepens.

Hypotony.

Red glow not clear.

Cortex not aspirating easily. The vitreous strands bring

the anterior and posterior capsule close to each other. And then it becomes difficult to aspirate the cortex.

➢ Vitreous movements and fluid, visco or air behind the capsule indicates posterior capsular tear.

If piece or fragment in posterior vitreous; put PCIOL in ciliary sulcus; close incision and send the patient to vitreoretinal surgeon. Sometimes in case vitreo retinal surgeon is not available, e.g. in periphery or patient is not willing or likely to go to retinal surgeon, then you have to manage on your own. Go down upto the piece with vitrectomy cutter and do vitrectomy anterior to fragment. Then start the irrigation with 20 gauge cannula. Take care that the incision is wide open and fluid can come out easily. Valve type incision does not allow the fragment to come out. So make a large incision. Keep it open. Fragment will come with the irrigating fluid into the anterior chamber.

If rent in posterior capsule is there, even then you can put PMMA lens or acrylic hydrophobic foldable lens on the anterior capsule, in the ciliary sulcus. This acrylic hydrophobic foldable PCIOL is preferred, as it unfolds little slowly and more controlled so you are sure that first haptic is in ciliary sulcus.

➢ Silicon IOL unfolds very fast and uncontrolled so rarely it may go through the rent in the vitreous and hence not preferred in such cases, where there is a rent in posterior capsule.

WHAT IS THE SECRET OF SUCCESS ?
"TO GET UP WHEN WE FALL DOWN"

When I make aspiration on, preset vacuum is achieved even though the tip is not visibly occluded. What is the problem?

If you press the footswitch and make the aspiration on then preset vacuum is achieved though any lens matter does not occlude tip. This indicates that there is block in aspiration line. Take out the handpiece and then put priming chamber. Adjust preset vacuum to nearly 500 and make phaco on. If there is some remnant of nucleus in the phaco needle it gets aspirated and block gets relieved. But still the preset vacuum is achieved then problem is there at tubing level. Like kink in the tube or lens matter somewhere clogging the tube. Take out the aspiration tube from the handpiece and deep in saline. Now make aspiration on by pressing footswitch. If the preset vacuum is reached then block is there in the tube or else in the handpiece including the needle.

Preset vacuum is not reached even though the aspiration is on and tip is occluded. Where is the problem?

Usually there is leak in the aspiration line, like aspiration tubing not firmly attached to handpiece. Another reason can be, in the machine where the peristaltic pump beads are not firmly pressing over the tube. For this change the tube on pump or put it firmly on the beads. Lock it properly.

My phaco tip is not getting tuned properly. Even if I press the footswitch completely I am not getting power. What is the problem?

Then mostly the needle is not fitting properly. Tighten it. Change it if necessary. If still tuning is not possible then the problem is in the handpiece itself.

If my phaco machine has too many surges, is it not a good machine? What should I do?

Every body talks about this. But we can demonstrate it to the phaco engineer if it is so. Apply priming chamber filled with the Ringer lactate. (see page 75, chapter 5). Then set the vacuum to routine required vacuum. This way, instead of talking too much, practically demonstrating the surge motivates the engineer to improve the machine fluidics. Surge can be more if there is air in the aspirating line. Take out this air.

My phaco machine has less phaco power. What should I do?

Phaco power is an important thing. You should be able to use other supportive maneuvers. If you want to engulf any quadrant then you can push the quadrant mechanically into the tip by chopper. This way with less energy also you can aspirate the quadrant.

Vent not proper (see page 78).

WE CAN NOT DIRECT THE WIND BUT WE CAN ADJUST OUR SAILS

It is even difficult to measure IOP by Schiøtz tonometer under topical anesthesia and you say that surgery is possible under topical?

Phaco beginners usually worry about movements of eyeball under topical anesthesia. On operation table when we are not operating and ask the patient to look up and down, he can do it. However, when we are operating, we are holding eyeball with two instruments. With chopper from side port and with phaco handpiece from main incision, it is impossible for the patient to move the eyeball in this situation as this two-instrument snuggly fix the eyeball.

Effect of topical anesthesia lasts longer on cornea than on conjunctiva. Touching conjunctiva is painful and it should be avoided. Lid movements are taken care of by speculum.

Normally we use pinky or super pinky to lower IOP in extracapsular cataract extraction. Here in phaco we do not use any other means to lower the IOP. Why is it so?

The basic concept of phaco rests upon closed chamber surgery. In extracapsular cataract extraction pressure in the anterior chamber almost equals to the atmospheric pressure. In this situation, we need to keep vitreous pressure at a lower level so that it does not push the posterior capsule and vitreous forward. To achieve this vitreous pressure is reduced by pinky or super pinky.

In closed chamber surgery like phaco, we increase the pressure in anterior chamber. (It is equivalent to height of the irrigation bottle). This pushes posterior capsule and vitreous behind. Thus, in closed chamber phaco surgery the anterior chamber pressure is increased. This pushes the posterior capsule and vitreous back.

In closed chamber surgery an additional advantage is that even if you rupture posterior capsule, vitreous may not come out if irrigating fluid does not enter the vitreous. The pressure in the anterior chamber pushes the vitreous back.

Thus, managing vitreous is easier in closed chamber surgery, even if there is rent in posterior capsule. However, one major disadvantage of closed chamber surgery is that nucleus drop can occur, which we never encountered previously in conventional extracapsular cataract extraction.

THE MAN WHO MAKES NO MISTAKES DOES NOT USUALLY MAKE ANYTHING

How to detect rent in posterior capsule that has occurred while doing hydrodissection?

There are certain alarming signs. You get a 'Click' sound and chamber, which was shallow, earlier, becomes deep automatically.

You try to hold the nucleus. Anterior chamber becomes irregular and nucleus becomes mobile. If this happens give the block and convert to routine extracapsular cataract extraction. While doing this, anterior chamber pressure should always be kept low, so that nucleus does not get pushed into vitreous. For pressing over the lower lip of incision and enlarging the incision you can do as indicated below:

Signs

Anterior chamber suddenly deepens

Hypotony.

Nucleus not rotating freely.

Red glow not clear.

Cortex not aspirating easily.

Sound of phaco changes if vitreous is touching the tip

Vitreous movements and fluid, visco or air behind the capsule indicates posterior capsular tear.

In case posterior capsule ruptures

The management depends on the stage at which rent has occurred (Flow Chart 8.2).

Few points are to be remembered while converting to extracapsular surgery. Don't try for new things at this stage. If you are on temporal side you can convert from 12 o'clock position. Extend the incision in such a way that it does not increaase the anterior chamber pressure at any time. If this happens then nucleus may go down. Extending the incision will reduce the pressure in anterior chamber and prevent the nucleus from sinking down.

What to do if rent in posterior capsule occurs while doing phaco and nuclear fragments are still remaining to be removed?

If you are in a learning phase, stop doing phaco (give block if under topical) and convert to routine extracapsular cataract extraction. For phaco learners it is always advisable to take superior rectus suture at the beginning of surgery. Once the posterior capsule ruptures, it is difficult to take this suture. It is always preferred to do extracapsular cataract extraction from headend side like you do routinely

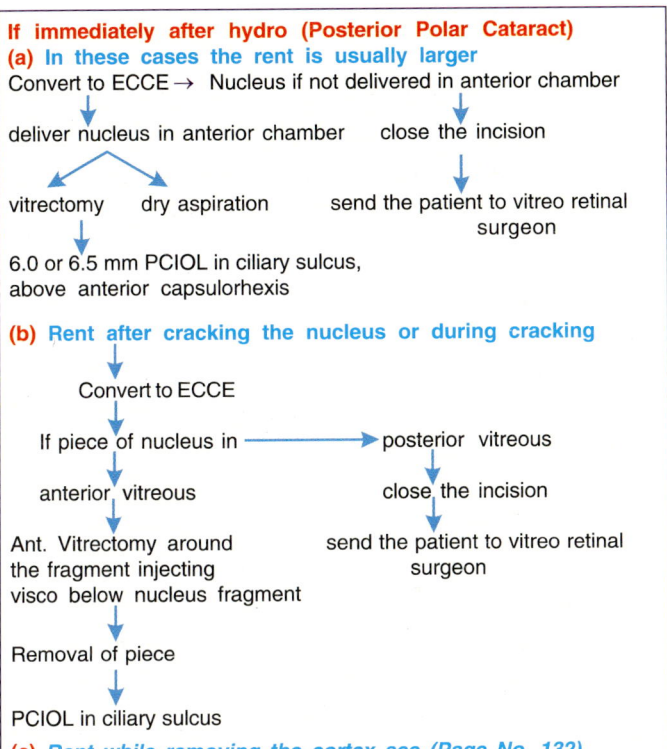

If immediately after hydro (Posterior Polar Cataract)
(a) In these cases the rent is usually larger
Convert to ECCE → Nucleus if not delivered in anterior chamber

deliver nucleus in anterior chamber   close the incision

vitrectomy   dry aspiration   send the patient to vitreo retinal
                                              surgeon

6.0 or 6.5 mm PCIOL in ciliary sulcus,
above anterior capsulorhexis

(b) Rent after cracking the nucleus or during cracking

Convert to ECCE

If piece of nucleus in ⟶ posterior vitreous

anterior vitreous   close the incision

Ant. Vitrectomy around   send the patient to vitreo retinal
the fragment injecting   surgeon
visco below nucleus fragment

Removal of piece

PCIOL in ciliary sulcus

(c) Rent while removing the cortex see (Page No. 132)

Flow Chart 8.2: Stagewise management of
rent in posterior capsule

ABOUT THE NUCLEUS DROP:
EVERYTIME I DID WELL AND
THAT I HEARD NEVER
ONCE I DID BAD AND THAT
I HEARD FOREVER

because we are well trained in it. Avoid doing any new things or maneuvers when posterior capsular rent is there. The phaco incision seals on automatically. If it leaks then it can be sutured with absorbable 10 zero polygalactin. Take care that while doing this, nucleus fragment does not go down in vitreous. Do not allow the anterior chamber pressure to rise. If this happens then enlarge the main phaco incision so that the wound does not remain a closed chamber wound but gets converted to open chamber like a conventional extracapsular cataract extraction wound. Remember that nucleus will sink in vitreous only when pressure in the anterior chamber is more than vitreous pressure. We can very well prevent this by converting closed chamber to open by enlarging the incision. Again you have to be careful that while enlarging the incision you should not allow the pressure in anterior chamber to rise. Take out viscoelastics from anterior chamber by pressing over the posterior lip of the incision.

What to do if rent in posterior capsule occurs when only cortical matter is present and nucleus has been completely removed?

Do close chamber vitrectomy with no or less irrigation. Make another side port incision. Through this vitrectomy can be done. Do bimanual irrigation aspiration with closed chamber. Cortex aspiration is easy with this procedure, as it is a closed chamber aspiration. Put IOL in the bag or on anterior capsule.

What to do if nuclear fragments or nucleus is in anterior one-third of vitreous?

Give block. Do routine extracapsular cataract extraction and remove nucleus as discussed earlier.

If nucleus or its fragments travel posteriorly in the vitreous, abandon the procedure. Take help of vitreo-retinal surgeon if possible immediately. If not, then put the IOL on anterior capsule, if that is possible, easily. Close the wound. Put the patient on higher dose of steroids. Inform relatives and patient that the part of cataract is inside (about the mishap). Although I know it is much embarrassing to inform patient about this. But it will add fuel to the fire if relatives of patient get this information from other eye specialist. To avoid even more embarrassing situation afterwards it is better to inform the patient before hand.

> SKILLS AREN'T ENOUGH.
> ITS YOUR ATTITUDE THAT
> MAKES THE DIFFERENCE

What should I do if there is leak from side port or main incision?

Let us first see the causes of leakage.

1. Large side port
2. Large main incision.
3. If your chopper or phaco tip is pressing firmly on one side or scleral lip of incision.

If the incision is large then it is always better to give a suture to the leaking side port or main incision. Then shift to a new incision as well as side port and proceed further. You may have to change the siting position also.

But if only side port is leaking, one can try and occlude the side port by cortical material itself and proceed further. Sometimes, this may happen automatically. The cortical mater comes with the fluid and blocks the side port.

The advantage of this is that it allows passage and movement of instruments through the side port but does not allow the fluid to come out.

If your chopper or phaco tip is pressing on scleral lip or one side of the wound then there will be more leakage from the wound. In this the surgeon should learn the technique to move the instruments inside the anterior chamber without pressing the lips of the wound. This can be learnt easily on goats' eye.

Why posterior capsule doesn't get ruptured easily in a close chamber (phaco) surgery?

In open chamber surgery like extracapsular cataract extraction, the capsule is bulging forward most of the time. This happens because pressure behind the capsule (vitreous pressure) is more than the pressure in anterior chamber. This bulging capsule is like a tense balloon that is prone for rupture even if touched by any sharp object. This is how chances of rent in the posterior capsule are more in routine extracapsular cataract surgery.

As against this, phaco is a closed chamber surgery, where the posterior capsule remains concave. Even if you touch it with a sharp object, there are less chances of getting rent. This is because the pressure in anterior chamber and vitreous pressure are equivalent. This minimizes chances of capsular rent.

What should be the ideal patient for phaco beginners?

There are so many criteria but if you want to see the all in one case then it is impossible to get the ideal case for phaco. You will never be able to operate. But following will be the criteria.

1. Chamber slightly on deeper side
2. Pupil fully dialates
3. Cornea bright
4. Anterior young patient so that zonules are not weak
5. No pseudo exfoliation
6. Grade II or III nucleus not very soft also
7. Not a posterior capsular cataract
8. A cooperative patient (a patient who shall not sue you for your mistakes).

If fluid is getting collected in the conjunctival sac and hampering visibility, what should be done?

1. Change the position of the patient's head. Tilt it slightly so that fluid drains out easily through the lateral canthus.
2. Do lateral canthotomy so that fluid drains out easily.

If conjunctival ballooning occurs and then fluid accumulates in the conjunctival sac and obscures the vision, what should be done?

To avoid this, corneal incision should not extend towards the conjunctiva. But if it happens, enlarge the conjunctival incision and retract the conjunctiva from the incision site. Now the conjunctival cut is away from the main phaco incision so the fluid does not pass below conjunctiva. With this the fluid shall not penetrate and balloon the conjunctiva (Fig. 8.2). If ballooning of conjunctiva is disturbing then retract the conjunctiva as above. Then squeeze the fluid out from the sub-conjunctival tissue by pressing with blunt spatula or muscle hook. You can incise over the most bulging part of conjunctiva. This will flatten the conjunctiva (Fig. 8.3).

If visibility is poor due to lipid secretion accumulating on cornea, what to do?

Put hydroxymethylcellulose on cornea and wash thoroughly. This washes out the secretions and visibility increases.

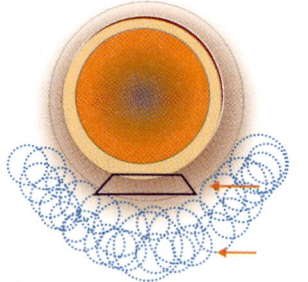

Clear corneal incision but corners extending towards conjunctival side

Ballooning of conjunctiva

Fig. 8.2: Shows how the edges of the corneal incision go towards the conjunctiva. This causes the fluid to enter in the conjunctiva, because of high pressure. This will lead to ballooning of the conjunctiva

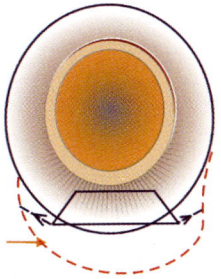

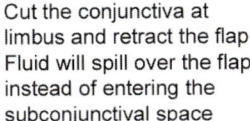
Cut the conjunctiva at limbus and retract the flap. Fluid will spill over the flap instead of entering the subconjunctival space

Fig. 8.3: Shows how giving the cut to the conjunctiva retracts the flap. This will drain the fluid. Also the fresh coming fluid will spill over this flap and prevent further ballooning

How to remove air bubbles, which are present in anterior chamber and obscure the view?

Let us first look into its causes—

Air bubbles can accumulate if phaco power is very high or anterior chamber has a tendency to collapse due to large side port incision. This sucks the atmospheric air inside.

Air bubbles can also come from irrigating fluid. To prevent this keep airway site in irrigating bottle away from the irrigating port (Fig. 8.4). Also a long needle like spinal needle can be used as airway. The tip of this needle passes above the fluid level in the bottle.

To manage air bubbles in anterior chamber –

a. Take out phaco handpiece. Now inject hydroxypropyl methylcellulose behind the bubble in such a way so as to push the bubble towards the incision. Simultaneously press the scleral lip, so that the bubble comes out along with the out coming fluid.

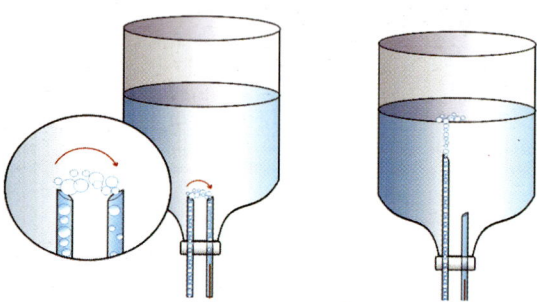

Fig. 8.4: Shows how the arrangement of the irrigating cannula and air needle should be in the bottle. If they are at same level then the air bubbles from airway cannula will enter the irrigating cannula. Hence the tip of the airway cannula should pass above the fluid level in the empty space or at least not at the level of the irrigating cannula but above it

b. Try to aspirate air bubbles with phaco tip with aspiration on, of course taking care that phaco power does not get activated.

How to do phaco in posterior polar cataract?

How to identify posterior polar cataract?

On slit lamp examination we can see a typical *onion pearl* appearance (Fig. 8.5) at the posterior pole. Patient is usually young below 40 years. Many times there is a pre-existing rent in the posterior capsule, which causes such type of cataract. Also, sometimes, on thorough examination one can see fine cortical particles suspended in the vitreous which floats with movement of eye. This is termed as fishtail appearance. It indicates that there is preexisting rent in posterior capsule.

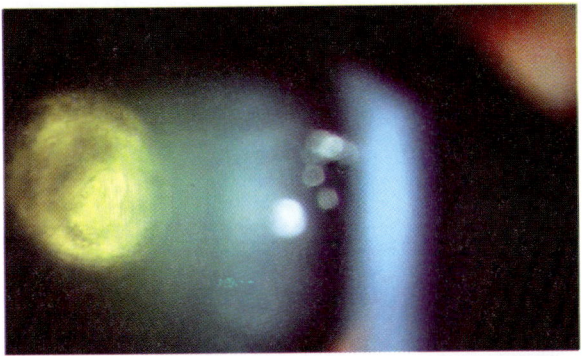

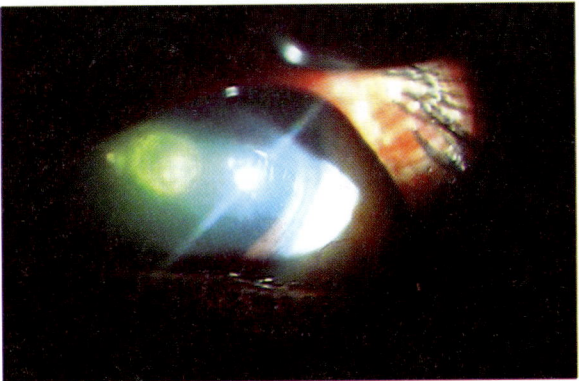

Fig. 8.5: Shows the typical onion pearl appearance
of the posterior polar cataract

This cataract should be differentiated from posterior
subcapsular cataract. On slitlamp examination you can
see opacity little bit inside posterior capsule. If you
are in dilemma then operate this like posterior polar
cataract.

Some special precautions

The first and foremost is *not to do hydrodissection. This may cause rent in posterior capsule and sinking of nucleus in vitreous. Do hydrodelineation* where the epinucleus is separated from central compact endonucleus by pushing balanced salt solution with the help of hydrodelineation cannula.

Technique: Pass a 25 or 26 no. cannula in the nucleus, as soon as it hits the endonucleus direction of the cannula is changed. Now pass the cannula tangential to the endonucleus , and a to-and-fro movement of the cannula is made to create a tract within the nucleus. Now the cannula is slightly retracted back to create a empty track. Now the fluid is gently but steadily pushed in the empty tract, which passes without much resistance, separating the epinucleus from the endonucleus. Often a circumferential golden ring is seen which outlines the cleavage between epinucleus and endonucleus.

While doing phaco, the machine parameters are kept at low level, i.e. low vacuum, low power and low flow rate. This is so because, if at all there is a preexisting rent in the posterior capsule, low machine parameters will prevent the rent from enlarging. Any turbulence in anterior chamber or sudden collapse of chamber can enlarge the rent. So avoid this. Now the nucleus and cortical mater is aspirated. The central opaque cortex should be removed at the end.

Soft nucleus

Phaco machine parameters

Keep the vacuum and power at low levels. Flow rate regular.

Exposed part of the tip is small. Like an ice cream, scoop out the central part, usually suction, but if not then use minimal phaco power, aspirates it. Go on doing this till you feel that small saucer shaped epinucleus is remaining.

Remove the handpiece out of anterior chamber. The anterior chamber collapses. Saucer shaped nucleus and epinucleus usually prolapses in the anterior chamber. Then aspirate it with phaco handpiece. Use of minimal power does not damage the cornea. If the epinucelus does not prolapse then push the visco behind the epinucleus and bring it into the anterior chamber. Now aspirate it.

Still if it is not prolapsing then do the hydrodissection and bring the epinuclear plate into anterior chamber.

In spite of all the procedures mentioned above the epinucleus is not prolapsing into the anterior chamber then go for sculpting of the epinucleus like ice-cream scoop. It has not prolapsed into the anterior chamber means it is thick and there is no danger of touching the posterior capsule by the tip. Again try the above mentioned procedure to bring the nucleus in anterior chamber. Bring it into pupillary plane or even into anterior chamber and then aspirate it with minimal phaco power. Don't worry, as power required be very less it will not cause any endothelial damage.

How to do phaco on last piece of nucleus so as to avoid rent in post capsule?

1. Phaco needle should be less exposed (Fig. 8.6). For this rotate the sleeve forward so that less part of phaco needle is exposed.
2. Reduce the vacuum and flow rate.
3. There should not be any leakage from the side port. This helps in reducing the surge. Take out the chopper from the side port. If small leak is there, then wait. Cortical matter or very tiny nucleus fragment will usually block the side port.
4. Rotate the phaco sleeve in such a manner that the irrigation port is facing towards the posterior capsule. Of course one opening shall be towards the corneal endothelium. You have to take care that this position is not there for a long time. But the advantage is that small surge will not allow the capsule to come in contact with the phaco tip as irrigation port is towards the posterior capsule. The irrigating fluid will move capsule away from the tip.

My microscope is not very good so I cannot learn Phaco!

It is always better to have very good microscope. But it is not essential to have the best. You can learn with ordinary microscope too. The problem you face is during capsulorhexis. But today you can use trypan blue. With this the capsule is stained and it becomes very easy to do capsulorhexis.

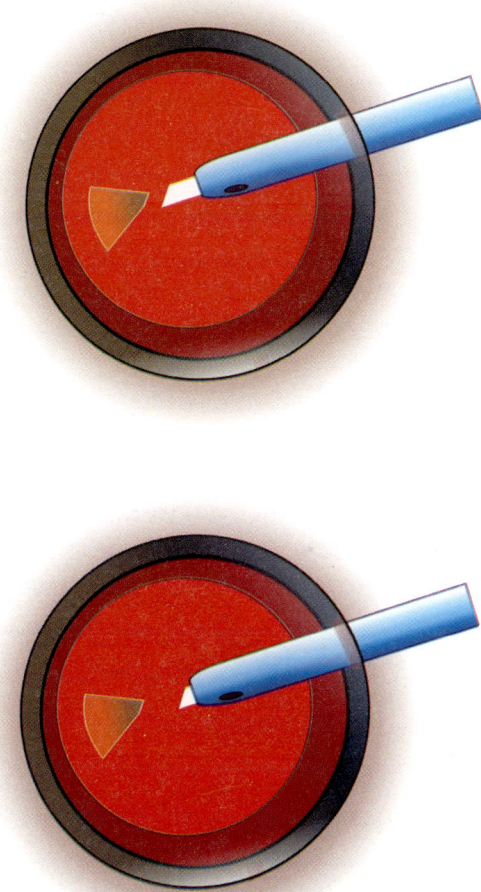

Fig. 8.6: Shows how the exposed part of the phaco needle is reduced while aspirating the last fragment

Use less magnification while operating—say around 6 in most of the phaco maneuvers. This has two advantages. First, the field of vision is more so you can see the more part of instruments. This increases control over the maneuvers. Secondly, the depth of focus is more so you can see cornea and posterior capsule at one time.

Increased magnification is required when you do capsulorhexis. The red glow should be maximum while doing capsulorhexis. This can be achieved by rotating the eye slightly nasally. This nasal rotation of eyeball is easier in temporal incision.

Increased magnification is used when you want to see that your IOL is in the bag or not. Similarly, while operating when you want to see the things clearly, you can increase the magnification see what you want to see. Then lower the magnification now you will be able to appreciate the same thing in lower magnification too. Now continue to operate in lower magnification. Another step to increase the magnification is to put hydroxypropyl methylcellulose drop on cornea, this acts as a lens and magnifies the structures temporarily without compromising field of vision.

What is chattering? How to avoid it?

Chattering means—when the nucleus fragment is near the tip and as phaco power is made on then the fragment, instead of getting emulsified and sucked in it, moves to-and-fro from tip. It moves away from tip and again gets attracted towards tip. Chattering may occur due to following reasons.

1. If tip is not occluded fully by nucleus fragment. Here the vacuum will not be built up. So there is no proper hold. So to get tip occluded increase the flow rate. This will bring the fragment close to the tip and tip will get occluded (Fig. 8.7).

2. If it is occurring even if the tip is occluded by fragment. Then two things are possible—vacuum is less (Fig. 8.8) or rarely phaco power used is very high.

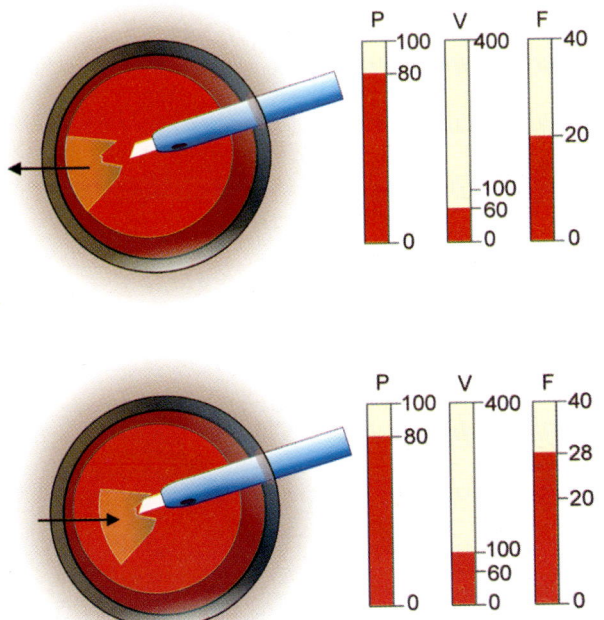

Fig. 8.7: Shows how chattering occurs due to low flow rate. If the flow rate is increased the flow of the fluid will push the fragment towards the phaco probe

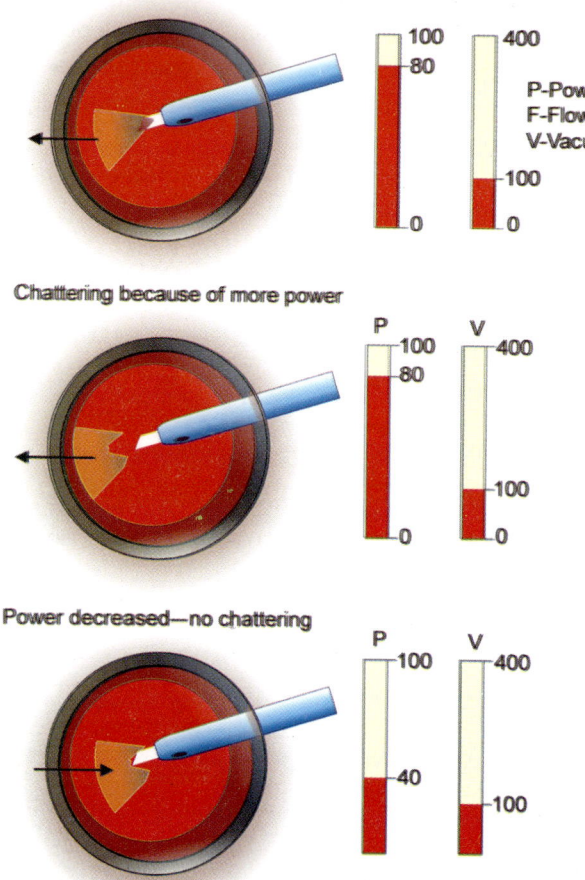

P-Power
F-Flow rate
V-Vacuum

Chattering because of more power

Power decreased—no chattering

Fig. 8.8: Shows how chattering occurs due to more phaco power used for last fragment. Decrease the power and aspirate the last fragment

How to put an IOL in the bag? (5.2 mm IOL)

Increase the incision to 5.1 mm or slightly more. This can be done by blade direction towards center of cornea. The direction should not be posteriorly. The posterior part of blade should press over the scleral lip while making the incision. If incision is made this way then the valve function is good. But, if direction of blade is towards the iris then the incision is likely to leak, as the lower flap hangs down.

Hold the lens with Liberman microring lens holding forceps. This has good grip because of circle at the end. Hold the lens at the edge. Insert the lens directing towards opposite limbus. Once the 60 percent of optic is in then change the direction of lens vertically down, that is, around 80 degrees vertical. The haptic should rub over the posterior capsule. The first loupe should go in the bag. Release the lens with loupe in the bag. Deepen the chamber with methylcellulose. Then with the dialer push the lens posteriorly, towards opposite clock position and dial. When it moves through 90 degrees then start pulling it towards incision, simultaneously pushing the lens posteriorly and dialing. In one stroke usually it will be in the bag. Maintain anterior chamber throughout the maneuver. If you do not maintain the chamber then it is difficult to put it in the bag. If it is difficult to maintain the chamber and the visco is coming out while maneuvering then take one suture and then dial. This can be practiced easily on goats eye.

Why to use 5.2 mm lens?

The material of foldable is not time tested as non-foldable usual PMMA lens. The cost is prohibitive. Those which are affordable, like hydrophilic foldable lenses, there are rare chances of deposits. In few it is difficult to do yag-capsulotomy. In India we get many hypermature cataract cases and in these patients posterior capsule is thick and opaque on operation table itself. So, even if lens may not allow the posterior capsule opacification but the existing we have to treat with YAG. Posterior capsulorhexis we do not want to do in old age so that the complication of cystoid macular edema or rarely anterior uveitis, if occurs, may spread posteriorly. In Indian eyes the pupil in old age is not more than 4 mm in most cases. This may be not true for western countries. So there are no chances of glare in night hours. Preoperative astigmatism in 80 percent of cases is around 1 diapter. If we take incision in steeper meridian, then preexisting astigmatism gets neutralized first. So ultimately you get very less astigmatism by 5.1 mm incision.

When using 5.2 mm PCIOL, irrigation aspiration should be done by Simcoe cannula. If we use routine automated irrigation aspiration handpiece, then the incision is not closed chamber incision. The fluid will leak from the sides of the instrument. This is the reason why irrigation aspiration done by Simcoe is better.

How to learn on goat's eyes? Why is it necessary?

We are following a programme of phaco training in our institution and in that learning on goat's eye is important step, which helps all surgeons to master the art quickly. He masters his reflexes. By repeatedly doing it he stores it in action memory. He can do it easily on patient's eye afterwards. The surgeon is more confident while doing surgery on patient's eye.

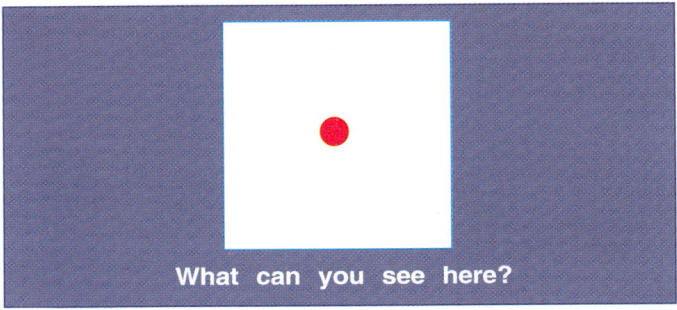

What can you see here?

Most of us see only the small black dot; but forget the large white area around. Black dot is like hands on training on patients, while the large white area represents ample opportunity to learn on goat's eyeball.

Why is it necessary to learn on goat's eyes?

While learning any new surgical technique we are afraid of it. It is but natural. In phaco surgery this phobia is even more. Not only to those who want to learn phaco, but to all those surgeons who want to learn cataract surgery. Practicing on goat's eyes is very helpful. There are many differences in surgical feel of goat's eye and human eye. But what we learn is how to adjust our posture and how to rest our fingers in temporal clear corneal incision (Fig. 8.9). Get accustomed to different steps till they are carried out at subconscious level. The same steps, when you carry

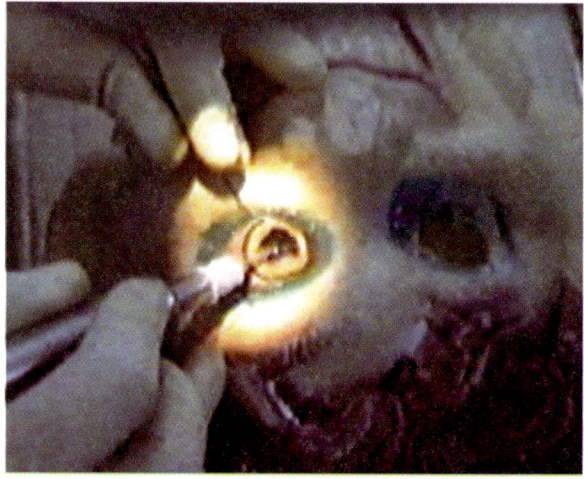

Fig. 8.9: Shows how the hands and fingers are rested

out on patients, you do not have to think over. You can get time to think and act on difficult steps when you operate on patients. Concentrate more on what can be learnt on goat's eye, than what is not possible.

For fixing the goat's eye we prepare the face mask. Pick up any face mask (which is available in *holi easily*) (Fig. 8.10) of size of normal face. Then melted wax is put in it (Fig. 8.11). Two small 3 ml hydroxymethylcellulose bottles are put at the place of eyes (Fig. 8.12). This gives place to fix eyeball (Fig. 8.13). The advantage of this is that the surgeon learns to rest his fingers and hands while working from temporal side.

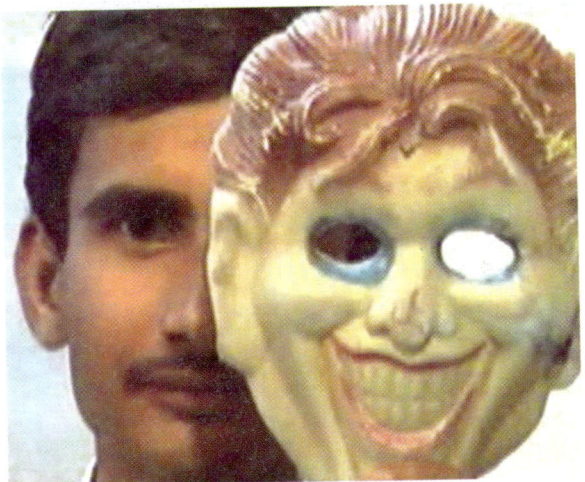

Fig. 8.10: Shows the face mask used

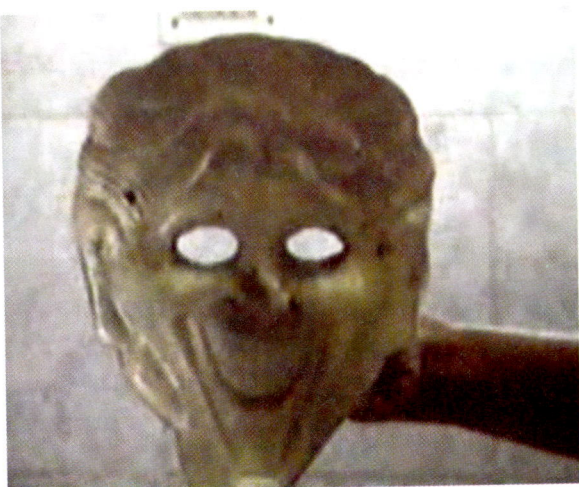

Fig. 8.11: Shows how melted wax is put in the mask

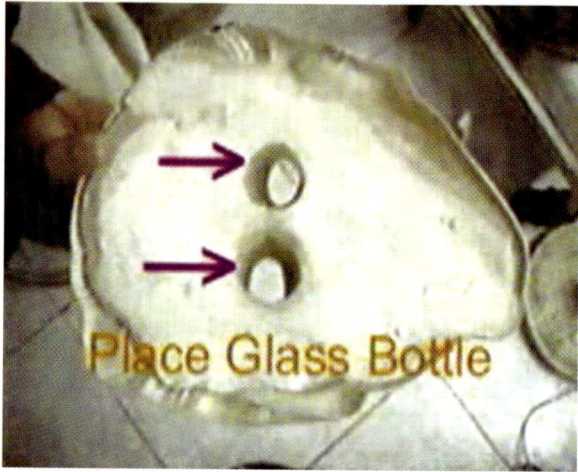

Fig. 8.12: Shows how glass bottles are placed, so we get two openings corresponding to orbital sockets

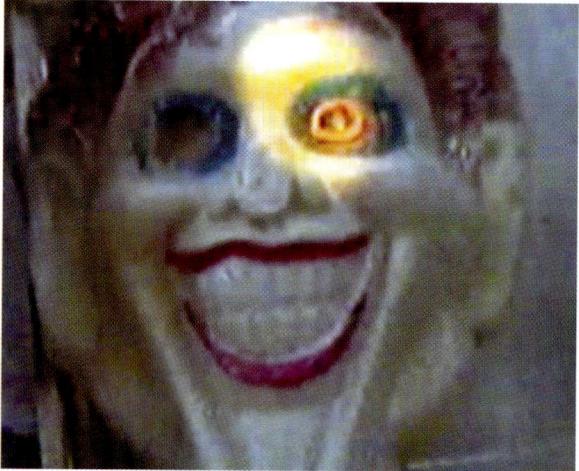

Fig. 8.13: Shows how the goat's eye is fixed into the mask

The different things which you can learn are given below:

1. You get accustomed with the depth perception.
2. You get accustomed to the handling of instruments in comparatively less field of vision, but with swiftness.
3. You can become friendly with your instruments and phaco machine. Build reflexes for the footswitch and different maneuvers.
4. To learn side port, feel for toughness of the eyeball. If eyeball is soft then inject viscoelastics from behind through optic nerve or air will also do. Once the eye ball is tense then choose the site for side port. The site should be 2 mm inside limbus so iris does not come in the way. Then with 20 gauge needle make a side port. Here you should learn to stabilize the globe with a swab stick. Also you should learn how to hold the syringe of 20 gauge needle. Make a side port so that it should just enter the anterior chamber and should not damage the anterior capsule. Your side port should not be too large neither it should be too small. Learn how to rest your fingers.
5. To learn main incision hold the eyeball. Make corneal incision with 3.2 mm keratome (Fig. 8.14). Try and make a self-sealing incision. Here you should practice and know about how much to enter the corneal layers. Also you should learn to make the main incision 90 degrees away from side port. You should see where the tip of your keratome is pointing.

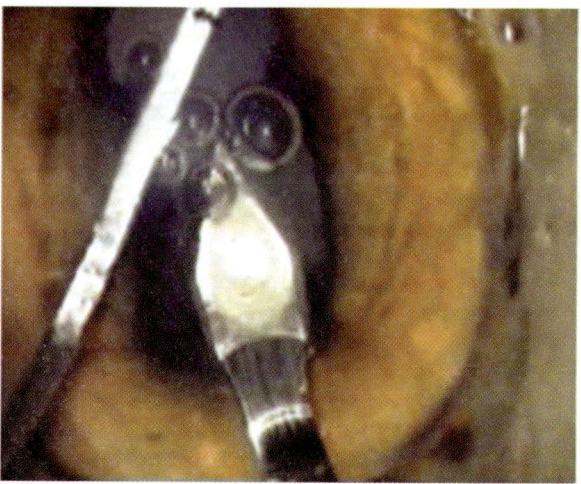

Fig. 8.14: Shows how the 3.2 tunnel is made. But you should not enter the keratome completely. And the tunnel should be about 1.5 mm inside the limbus

6. Capsulorhexis—the anterior capsule of goat's eye is tougher than human eye. Hence you get a false impression of the anterior capsule. Here what you have to learn is the movement of your fingers. How to hold the forceps and do the rhexis without allowing the anterior chamber to collapse. How the force should act, i.e. posteriorly and towards center. Also you can learn to extend the rhexis after giving a cut to the previous margin.

7. For phaco beginners, it is important to become friendly with their phaco machine, it's dynamics. How to change the parameters, how should be the tubing

connections? You should be very well versed with positions 1, 2 and 3 of the footpedal. Now your ears should know the different audible signals. You should spend time with your machine to know these audible signals and develop reflexes so that you don't have to think about it. The movement should occur reflexely. This will help in building up your confidence.

8. Start with your phaco. The nucleus extracted from the human eye, during the conventional ECCE or manual small incision cataract surgery, is inserted into the anterior chamber of goat's eye (Fig. 8.15). Learn to introduce the probe into anterior chamber. Now insert the chopper into anterior chamber. This is very important step in phaco. You should be able to introduce your chopper easily. Now learn to remove the chopper from anterior chamber with irrigation on, which is an equally important step. Here many beginners forget to keep the irrigation on and this makes removal of chopper difficult because the anterior chamber collapses as soon as you remove the probe. It is difficult to remove the chopper from shallow anterior chamber.

9. Once you have adjusted with above steps, start with your phaco. After occlusion of the probe with nucleus you hear a typical musical note. Here you should learn to hold the nucleus in position 2. Now insert your chopper in substance of the nucleus and give little phaco power. The nucleus of goat's eye is softer

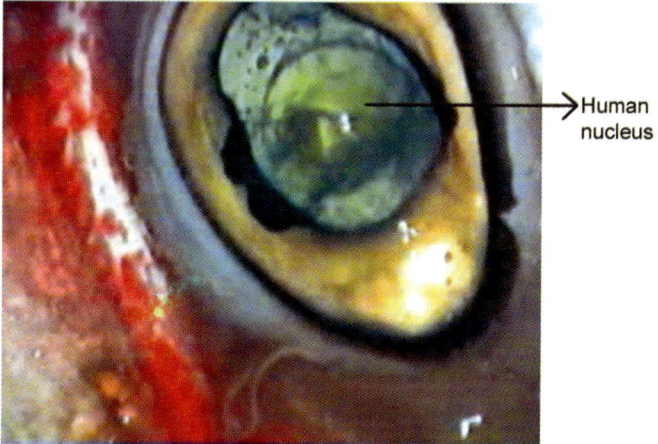

Fig. 8.15: Shows how human nucleus is placed into the anterior chamber of goat's eye

than human eye. The important steps here to learn are to hold the nucleus in position 2, and embed your chopper. Dialing the nucleus is another important step.

The nucleus of goat's eye is very soft. To overcome this problem the nucleus that was removed after ECCE surgery, is used. Make a 7 mm incision in corneal valve fashion and put this nucleus inside the goat's soft nucleus. The 7 mm incision is sutured (Fig. 8.16). Then make a fresh phaco incision on opposite side. Try cracking of nucleus (Fig. 8.17). So now it gives natural feel of dealing with nucleus.

10. After completing the phaco, one can learn 'how to insert the IOL in the bag'.

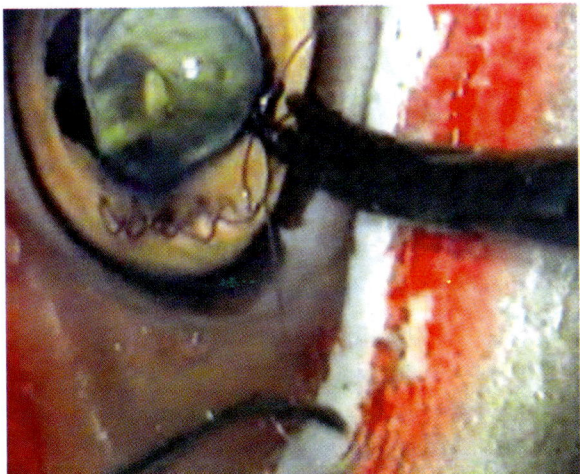

Fig. 8.16: Shows how the incision is sutured after placing the human nucleus

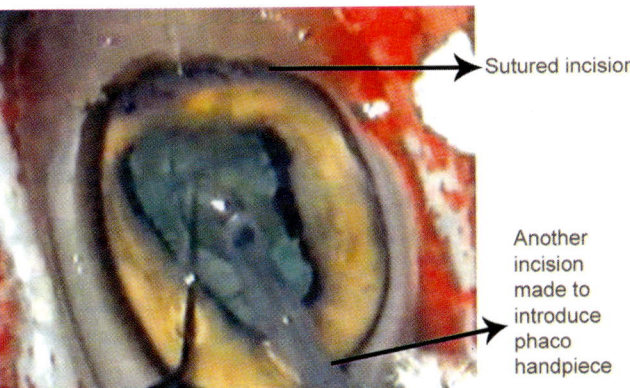

Sutured incision

Another incision made to introduce phaco handpiece

Fig. 8.17: Shows how phaco is tried on human nucleus put in goat's eye

How to shift over to topical?

If you think that you have mastered the phaco maneuvers and you can do it under peribulbar, then choose a patient for topical anesthesia. The criteria are same as for ideal phaco patient (see ideal patient for phaco). The pain tolerance should be above average.

There are certain precautions you have to take to avoid pain or discomfort to the patient. Do not touch conjunctiva. While doing side port incision fix the eyeball by using swab stick instead of forceps. If you want to fix or rotate the eye then insert instrument in the side port and move the eye. Rarely you can hold the lip of side port incision with Huskin's forceps when you have to hold the eye firmly.

The question peeps in mind is—if I want to convert to phaco under retrobulbar or routine extracapsular cataract extraction under peribulbar block? What if I land up in certain complications like rent in posterior capsule and I want to give infiltration anesthesia. How should I go ahead?

The conversion is simple. Push hydroxypropyl methylcellulose in anterior chamber. As the wound is self-sealing there will not be any leak now. Give block as per your routine way. If you want to put pressure on eye after this, then you can use any way, but in sterile conditions. As in the eye hydroxypropyl methylcellulose is there, the eyeball will not collapse. Then start surgery as per the case under infiltration anesthesia. You can take superior rectus suture also if you feel it necessary.

Why inflammation is less in phaco?

Minimal surgical trauma or no touch to iris. The substances that are released on touch cause inflammation. But as irrigation is there, it constantly washes out such substances.

Why infection is less?

Time required for experienced surgeon is less. Constantly fluid is coming out. No microorganisms can enter easily. Like in sterile drug manufacturing high pressure is there in the room so that there are less chances of micro-organisms entering the room. Similarly here the pressure in anterior chamber is high and fluid is constantly coming out.

Why use TUR set or irrigation tube of large bore?

If it is small bore then surge phenomenon shall be more. As fluid sucked out is replaced slowly if irrigation fluid tubings have small bore. So always use irrigation tubing of large bore and not of IV set. Prostrate surgeon or general surgeon for lavage uses TUR set which can be used here.

Which type of eye speculum is better for phaco surgery?

The one that you are accustomed to is the best one. But I am using routinely the universal eye speculum. Though it appears that it will press over the eyeball that is not true. It lifts up the lids away from the eyeball and does not press over the eye. If it is pressing over eyeball you can change to new one. Slight pressure over the eyeball does not do any harm in phaco, as it is closed chamber surgery.

The advantage is that exposure is better, lid retraction is better. If you are operating under topical even if patient wants to close the lids forcibly, he cannot. In topical anesthesia, if we use wire speculum then patient can squeeze the lids. This is not possible with universal eye speculum.

If palpebral aperture is small, what to do?

This becomes evident when the exposure is not complete, the cornea is covered by lids after applying the eye speculum. In this if you are doing it under topical, better to give block. This relaxes the muscles and you get more exposure. But if still the exposure is not good, then do lateral canthotomy.

Why should we use ice cold ringer lactate solution or balanced salt solution and hydroxypropyl methylcellulose?

It is always better to use ice cold ringer lactate solution chilled up to 4 to 6 degrees. It neutralizes heat produced by phaco tip. This may give protection against possible corneal burns. It also anesthetizes the conjunctiva to some extent.

The same thing is true for chilled hydroxypropyl methylcellulose, which becomes more viscous at this temperature.

Does viscosity of hydroxypropyl methylcellulose matter?

If the viscosity of methylcellulose is more it becomes more difficult to take it out at the end of the surgery. This may lead to inflammation postoperatively. That is why it is better to use methylcellulose of lower viscosity whenever highly viscous hydroxypropyl methylcellulose is not essential.

What to do in case of electricity failure while using phaco machine?

While doing Phaco it is necessary to have constant supply of electricity for Phaco machine and operating microscope. Though rarely, Phaco machine especially may create problems when it stops abruptly. Generators do not help in this situation as it takes few seconds to start. Uninterrupted power supply (UPS) used for computers are useful alternative for short duration till the generator takes over.

How to change settings of phaco machine while operating?

For changing the vacuum or other settings on control panel it is a good idea to place transparent sterile drape covering the control panel. This always helps to do all changes in settings even by a scrubbed associate rather than by any other unscrubbed person.

Newer machines nowadays come with foot-operated control panel.

What to do if the incision (tunnel) width is less?

While taking incision if you feel that incision width is smaller than desired, then move the blade upward while remaining within the corneal lamellae. This increases the width of incision. If entry of blade in anterior chamber is too early and you have not yet completed the incision, then there are two options. You can either abandon the incision or take a fresh incision at another site or keep the length of incision lesser than desired. Suppose you take 3.2 mm length regularly then you can take 3.1 mm in this case. Smaller the width of the incision, more is the fluid leak. To avoid this you can partly compensate by reducing length. If the blade is too sharp then the entry in anterior chamber may become too early and width will be less as compared to desired width. This is also true when eyeball is very tense or hard. The width of incision will be less than the desired incision.

If the width is small the advantage for the beginner is that maneuverability in anterior chamber is easy.

But there are distinct disadvantages like—more fluid is required as leak is more and secondly, you may need to suture the wound at the end.

If the incision width (tunnel width) is more, what to do?

Suppose you are in the midst of taking incision and you feel that width you will be getting is more, then change the direction of the blade abruptly, making it towards the optic nerve and enter the anterior chamber. If the sharpness of blade is less, you have more chances of getting more width of incision. If eyeball is soft, there are more chances of getting more width.

Suppose you get more width than that expected, then the problem anticipated would be like difficult maneuverability or getting more hydration of wound. When you move the phaco tip towards the incision, irrigation openings of the sleeve will be in wound and chamber may collapse.

EXCELLENCE CAN BE ATTAINED IF YOU ...
* CARE MORE THAN
  OTHERS THINK IS WISE
* RISK MORE THAN
  OTHERS THINK IS SAFE
* DREAM MORE THAN
  OTHERS THINK IS PRACTICAL
* EXPECT MORE THAN
  OTHERS THINK IS POSSIBLE

Chapter 9

Actions: They Speak for Themselves

We have discussed about action memory in earlier chapters. Usually we are doing even very important, skillful actions at subconscious level and reflexly most of the times, without feeling the stress of it. To develop these reflexes we have to practice a particular action several times. As far as mastering phaco is concerned, it is not possible to develop this reflex while learning on patients' eyes. It is desired to learn it on goats' eyes or eye-bank eyes or in presence of an experienced phaco surgeon.

This is not enough. You need to perform all these actions even in your imaginations repeatedly, visualize them often, as if you are actually doing it. This reduces the learning time to a great extent because you have visualized everything, as if you have performed that action several times before actually doing it.

Sometimes it so happens that you have mastered a particular action, but it is difficult to explain—how to do it. Just like riding a bicycle. You are a master in balancing on it but if somebody asks you to demonstrate the art of balancing in slow motion, you invariably fail. Doing phaco is similar to this. The procedure needs swiftness, you can't afford to be slow but at the same time you can't be very hasty either.

I am writing a big deal about actions. While reading about it you may develop a phobia about it, thinking that they are very difficult to perform. But in reality it is not so. Once you perform these actions two or three times, you start doing them automatically at a subconscious level. If you are not used to eating Chinese food with sticks, try it. Once you get used to it you never feel the stress of doing it.

Different surgeons adapt different actions as per their convenience. There is nothing like good action or bad action. Only remember that every person performs different actions.

Procedures to be followed whenever we want to insert the phaco tip inside the nucleus so as to embed it inside the nucleus.

Phaco tip should push the nucleus by 1 mm and not more. Otherwise there will be stretch on zonules. Then make phaco on. With this, phaco tip should go inside. If this fails to occur, increase the phaco power but avoid the temptation to push the phaco tip. The nucleus shall get attracted towards the phaco tip automatically. Sometimes, if the flow rate is less, then you may increase the flow rate to attract the nucleus towards the tip. Phaco tip should never be moved. If you support the nucleus by chopper just by touching the hard part of nucleus, this helps the tip to get embedded easily with less phaco power.

Additional Dimensions: Time and Speed (swiftness) in Surgery

In surgery, time should not be a major criteria. But, if you can do the surgery in minimal time, maintaining the quality, it is always beneficial to the patient and surgeon. The patient, if under topical, can cooperate for short duration and if surgical time prolongs then he may become restless and may not be able to cooperate.

We reduce the probability of infection and surgical trauma to the ocular structures if time taken for surgery is less, of course if other parameters are same. *(Of course other things remain same)*. I shall like to elaborate on this. Logically I feel that scleral tunnel is better procedure as compared to clear corneal incision as it reduces corneal endothelial damage. This is because the incision is away from the cornea. But when it comes to practice, things are different. Surgeon, who is well experienced in both—scleral tunnel as well as clear corneal—will be able to complete phaco with less Phaco time and less maneuvers in anterior chamber if the incision is clear corneal. In this way we can ultimately reduce the endothelial damage in clear corneal incision. Thus, time is important factor in surgery.

Some Prophylactic Measures

Irrespective of whether you need to give intravenous injections or not, intravenous line should be patent. Like intracath or scalp vein set should be fixed to the patient prior to surgery. This way we can manage the emergencies, if any. This is especially true for those who do not get services of a standby anesthetist routinely like surgeons working in peripheral area.

Pulse oximeter is a great asset in operation room and every theatre should be equipped with it. It can detect vasovagal attacks and respiratory depression in early period.

1. *Pyramid incision*—The advantage of pyramid incision is that maneuverability is better as compared to square incision. Even leaks are less, as inner lip is still smaller in size. Secondly, the pinching action of incision on the Phaco handpiece is less, as it is smaller in size only at the end (Fig. 9.1). This way movements of hand-piece can be made easily.

2. *Opening of the tip*—Hence fluid can not rush inside suddenly when the occlusion is released.

The aspiration bypass small hole in the phaco needle has the advantage that even if the tip is occluded the needle does not become hot as small amount of fluid is constantly aspirated which keeps the phaco needle cool. However, I feel that the disadvantage is, it gets broken easily at the site of hole and life of needle is less.

You should not press the reflux switch for long time as in some of the machine fluid, which comes, as reflux fluid

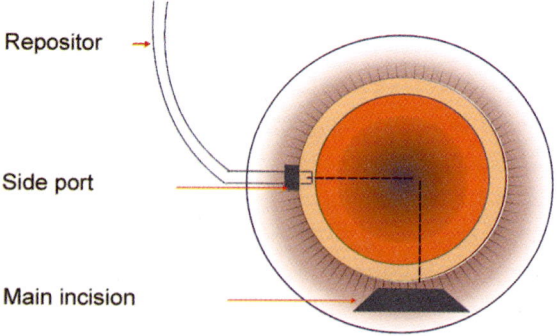

Fig. 9.1: Shows how the main incision should be, i.e. wedge shaped

is unsterile. If we press it for few seconds then it releases the iris or unwanted tissue that is caught accidentally. Refluxing the aspirated fluid does this. But if reflux switch is pressed for long time more amount of fluid is refluxed and which may be unsterile.

How to hold the eyeball?

While doing phacoemulsification it is essential to hold the eye in a particular position for doing all the maneuvers. This enhances the red glow and visibility and also offers stability that is necessary. There are different ways to do this. One way is to put iris repositor in side port incision, which gives some hold. In the direction, opposite to the side port, the patient can move the eye, especially if it is under topical anesthesia. If you are operating under block and still not satisfied with the stability, you can hold at limbus with Huskin's forceps. Another way is to hold with Huskin's forceps in such a way that one of the tongs is in side port incision whereas the other remains on the outer surface of cornea (Fig. 9.2).

How to insert and take out the chopper?

It is better to learn this technique on goat's eyeball.

While inserting the chopper, anterior chamber should be deep. To achieve this you can either use the visco-elastics or can keep the phaco tip in with irrigation on. Then insert the chopper in such a way that its flat surface is parallel to iris surface and the length of tip should be parallel to side port. And then rotate handle to make it vertical and at the same time push inside (Fig. 9.3).

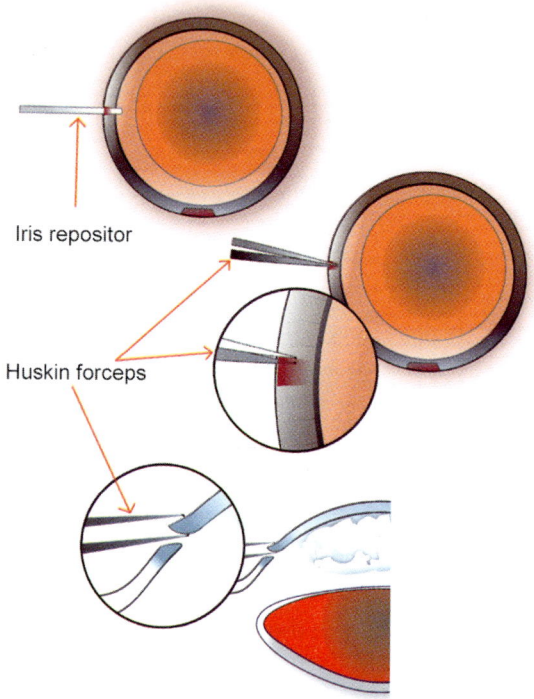

Iris repositor

Huskin forceps

Figs 9.2A and B: A. Shows iris repositor in the side port stabilizing the eyeball. **B.** Shows how the eyeball is held with the Huskin's forceps. One of the tongs is in the side port and the other is on the surface of the cornea

While removing the chopper also, anterior chamber should be deep. If phaco tip and chopper is in anterior chamber, one should remove the chopper first. Instead if the phaco tip is removed before chopper, it will cause collapse of anterior chamber. While removing the chopper irrigation should be on. Make the chopper parallel to iris

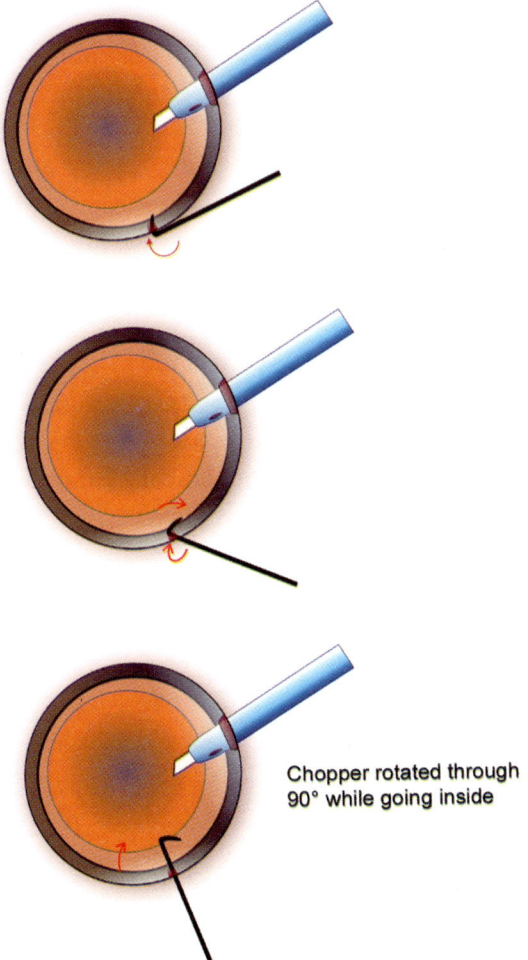

Chopper rotated through
90° while going inside

Fig. 9.3: Shows how to insert the chopper.
The direction of the movement of the chopper is shown

surface and then move handle in such a way that the length of tip is parallel to side port.

How to identify the site of side port and main incision?

Sometimes you feel as if the incisions are lost and you are unable to locate them. This is especially difficult for a beginner. Simple way to locate them is by spreading trypan blue with the help of cannula over the outer edge of incision, so that it becomes easy to identify the site due to its blue color. It is better that incision is slightly inside limbus.

While doing phaco in hard cataract I have landed up with thin plate of nucleus. I am afraid of touching the posterior capsule. How should I deal with the remaining plate?

While dividing the nucleus, crack must go through and through involving total depth as well as center of nucleus. If it is not done in this manner, you may come closer to the posterior capsule and there remains no thick and dense part of the nucleus that can be held firmly. What remains is, just a saucer shaped portion of the nucleus that is difficult to remove.

In such cases where a thin plate is remaining, it becomes difficult to embed the probe into the nucleus. Here, you can mechanically divide the nucleus with the help of dialer and probe. Alternatively you can push little visco below the plate, create some space for probe and then embed the probe into the nucleus. Pass the dialer below the plate. Now crack the plate. This will give you some space in the center. Then aspirate it using low phaco power.

Frequently asked questions related to different maneuvers and postures

How to take support while taking a side port incision?

Initially you may find it little difficult in first few cases but once you get used to it, you will say it is easiest to do. I will tell you the secret of doing it. You can have your own modifications later on. I give support to the eyeball by swab stick at a position opposite to the site of incision. This is especially necessary if you are operating under topical, for it shall be very painful, touching the conjunctiva. However, under peribulbar block you can hold the conjunctiva at limbus with Huskin's forceps (at position opposite to the site of incision). Now to make side port incision, take support of left hand if you are a right handed person. This is best learnt on goat's eyes and eye bank eyes.

How can we make ourselves comfortable while sitting on temporal side and manage to operate footswitch comfortably?

This can be done easily on goat's eye, fixed in a face mask as narrated earlier.

How to rotate the nucleus? (Fig. 9.4)

Before you try to rotate the nucleus, the prerequisites are that the anterior chamber should be deep and the

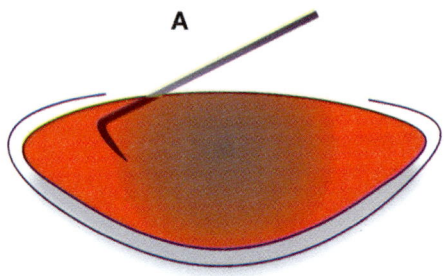

A

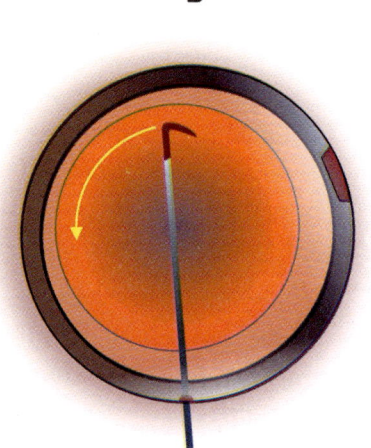

B

Fig. 9.4: Shows how to rotate the nucleus. The anterior chamber should be deep and try to rotate with the angle of the dialer rather than tip of the dialer. Here hydrodissection should be good enough

hydrodissection should be complete. Push hydroxypropyl methylcellulose in order to deepen the anterior chamber. Then the Sinsky hook enters from side port into an area of nucleus best suitable for rotation—the area that is not too soft; otherwise the dialer will pass through like cheese wire instead of rotating the nucleus. The simple way for this is to pass the dialer from periphery towards the center in oblique fashion (as if you want to dial). The dialer will cut through unless it meets with a hard part. At this point cutting action stops. Now you need to change the direction using force as if you are dialing. Give a little push posteriorly with the bent portion of the dialer. Do not hold the dialer in a vertical fashion. Deepen the anterior chamber whenever you feel it is shallow. If the nucleus is too soft then you can use mushroom dialer. This has small ballpoint; so instead of cutting through it will dial the nucleus.

How to polish the posterior capsule?

If you keep the vacuum less and move the irrigation aspiration tip over the capsule it removes the lens fibers that are adherent to the capsule.

But I still use Nightingale ring polisher, which is used in ECCE to polish the capsule. This has ring at the end, which acts like a scraper. When you see it you may feel that it will cause rent in posterior capsule. But, if you rub it over the capsule when the capsule is concave (Fig. 9.5A), then there are no chances of capsular tear. However, if you continue doing the procedure in a shallow anterior chamber, surface of the capsule becomes convex increasing chances of capsular rent (Fig. 9.5B). You should polish

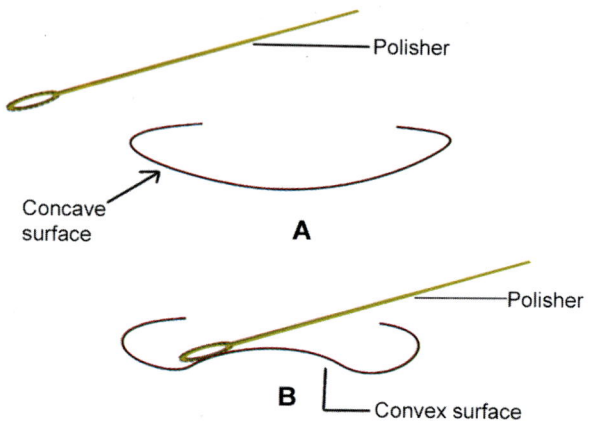

Figs 9.5A and B: A. Shows how polishing is done. The surface is concave here. As in deep anterior chamber in phaco surgery. **B.** Shows how the surface is convex, as in shallow anterior chamber, in ECCE

the equatorial region meticulously. This area contains more number of reduplicating cells. Polishing helps in removing these cells and even the lens fibers, which are present in this region.

How to seek finger rest when we are sitting on temporal side?

This can be learnt by doing routine ECCE (with small nucleus) from temporal side. In our institute we have prepared a facemask. We place goat's eye over the orbital region of facemask and operate from temporal side. With this you can learn to take proper position of hands giving rest to your fingers.

How to enhance the red glow?

Move the eye in such position that red glow shall be better. Usually moving nasally makes this clearer if surgeon is sitting on temporal side.

If visibility is poor what are the problems and remedies?

One has to look into its cause first. Let us see one by one.

Dry cornea: Put saline on the cornea or spread hydroxypropyl methylcellulose on the epithelial surface of cornea. Do not allow the cornea or hydroxypropyl methylcellulose on it to get dried up.

Trypan blue: Too much of trypan blue turns everything bluish and glow is hampered.

Oily substances: These may act like a froth hampering visibility. Put hydroxymethylcellulose on cornea and wash thoroughly. This washes out the secretions and visibility increases.

Edema of the corneal epithelium: It may be due to toxicity resulting from local eye drops or mild variety of dry eye. If it is disturbing too much then peel off epithelium by rubbing with swab stick.

Turbid viscoelastics: Hydroxypropyl methylcellulose may be turbid or less transparent. You can change the brand and choose a transparent one.

Air bubbles in anterior chamber: See page no. 137.

Problems with microscope: The problem may be in the

microscope like—no stereopsis or interpupillary distance may not be properly adjusted. When right eyepiece is focused, left is out of focus. Adjust the eyepiece by rotating it.

Hydroxypropyl methylcellulose or saline drops on the objective of microscope may also cause blurring. Clean with wet tissue paper dipped in distilled water.

Loose electricity fittings: Light cords may not have been fitted properly and snuggly. Bulb may not be at a proper place. Even if it is displaced slightly, light intensity shall go down.

How to insert the 5.2 mm IOL in the bag?

I use Liberman microring lens forceps to hold the intra-ocular lens. It is held near the optic haptic junction. The forceps, which can hold the lens at periphery, is better. If you hold the lens at center of optics then you need large incision to push the lens with forceps. So use Liberman ring forceps to hold the lens at periphery. Then I push it in the main incision, holding the eyeball by iris repositor, placed, in the side port. The direction of the force is in the direction of plane of incision (that is in iris plane). Of course, the loop should not touch the cornea. As soon as half of the optics is in, I turn the direction towards posterior capsule. Then I rub the loop against posterior capsule, and once the optic is in anterior chamber, I loosen my grip on lens.

How to dial the IOL?

This I think needs to be explained because I have seen

many times, we only go on dialing and the lens moves over the iris surface. It does not go in the bag. In this situation, I start dialing when one loop is inside and another is in incision. I push the dialer with its bent against the optic haptic junction. The force should push towards opposite side and posteriorly with dialing action. Once the dialing is over in a quarter of a circle, I start pulling the lens towards the incision and pushing it posteriorly with dialing. In most cases it is in the bag with the movements in three-quarters of a circle.

How to insert the chopper?

The anterior chamber should be deep. To achieve this, put irrigation on, keeping phaco tip inside. When the chopper is in anterior chamber, nucleus is firmly held in the phaco tip with vacuum achieved and phaco tip is embedded. Move the nucleus towards the incision by 1 mm. Now insert the chopper at the capsulorhexis border or even you can go below it. The question is—how to go below it without damaging the capsulorhexis? (Fig. 9.3). Hold the chopper in such a way that it's bent portion is towards the capsulorhexis border. Then traverse through the cortex below the border. Assess hardness of the nucleus by moving the chopper towards the center first and then move towards the periphery. Now if you want to embed it even deeper and then push it in such a way that it is feeding the nucleus in the phaco tip. This helps the vacuum.

How to hold the phaco handpiece?

Best way is to hold it like a pen, as we are accustomed to

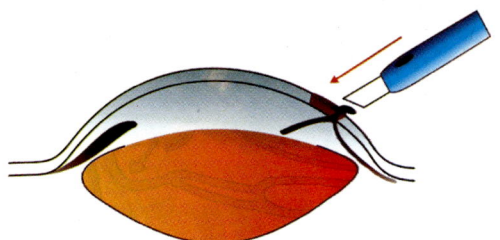

Fig. 9.6: Shows how phaco handpiece is inserted in cases of iris prolapse. The bevel is kept down while entering the anterior chamber. Routinely it is directed upwards

write and hold the instrument in this way and do manipulation in anterior chamber.

How to insert the phaco handpiece?

While inserting the phaco handpiece we should keep the bevel up. It is better to make irrigation on before inserting the handpiece in anterior chamber. The advantage is that when phaco tip is in the anterior chamber, you do not get air bubbles there. This is especially true for my machine. But if I feel the iris is coming in the way of phaco tip then I push the needle with bevel down after injecting hydroxypropyl methylcellulose from side port. This avoids touch of iris with phaco needle (Fig. 9.6).

What is the angle of bevel (of phaco needle)?

I routinely use 30 degree bevel needle for nearly all phaco cases (Fig. 9.7).

How to learn this wobbling technique (Fig. 9.8)

Basically you start this procedure while doing irrigation

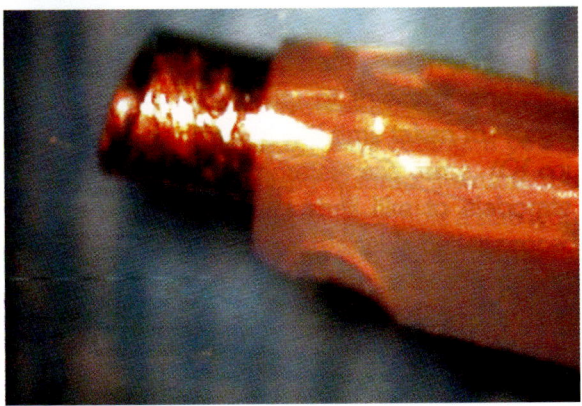

Fig. 9.7: Shows the tip of phaco handpiece.
The angle is about 30 degree

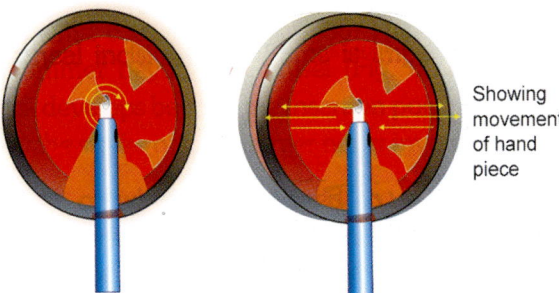

Showing
movement
of hand
piece

Fig. 9.8: Shows how the phaco handpiece is moved in the
anterior chamber. This is called "WOBBLING"

and aspiration. No other instrument should be inside the
anterior chamber or, in other words, only irrigation
aspiration handpiece should be in the anterior chamber.
Once the tip gets occluded then only rotation movement
is done swiftly but not hastily. This helps in fast aspiration

of the cortex. Once you master this technique with irrigation aspiration handpiece, you can try it with phaco tip. Only when the tip gets occluded, you are supposed to make circular movement swiftly. This will help in aspirating out the hard nucleus part.

How to learn to aspirate the subincisional cortex?

For aspirating the subincisional cortex, push hydroxypropyl methylcellulose to deepen the anterior chamber or the bag. Or else this hydroxypropyl methylcellulose should be injected in the bag before introducing the irrigation aspiration handpiece. Hold irrigation aspiration handpiece in a way that you will be able to rotate it inside the anterior chamber in such a fashion that the aspirating port is at the level of anterior capsule. This will never catch the posterior capsule and the subincisional cortex can be easily aspirated. Routinely we hold the handpiece like a pen with use of three fingers but when you want to rotate it for aspiration of subincisional cortex, the hold is slightly different. It is in four fingers so that you can rotate it when you want to. While rotating, see that only the irrigation is on. No aspiration is needed. Aspiration is on, only when the aspiration port is at the level of capsule.

Another method of aspirating the subincisional cortex is to take out the cortex from side port (Fig. 9.9).

By and large, for a soft nucleus settings of vacuum and phaco power are low. If you sculpt then the tip gets occluded partially. Preset vacuum is not achieved in this situation as the tip is partially occluded and it does not attract the nucleus.

Subincisional cortex removal

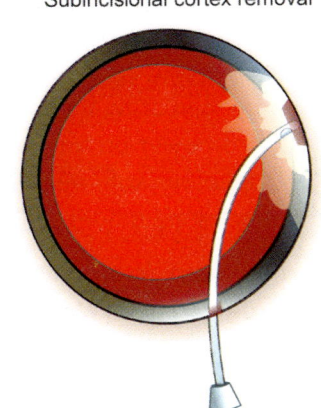

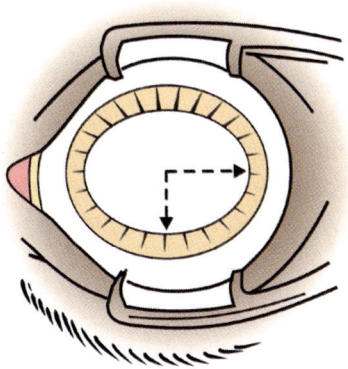

Fig. 9.9: Shows how subincisional cortex is aspirated

In such a situation bring the phaco tip in the center and make phaco on for fraction of seconds. This will aspirate the contents in the tip and relieve the partial block, which was hampering the proper functioning. Similarly, if you are near periphery then bring the phaco tip near the cortex and make phaco power on for fraction of second and this helps in attracting soft nucleus towards tip. Increasing the flow rate alone may not help.

When I am doing phaco from temporal side the eyeball moves nasally. What is the problem?

When the phaco beginner applies the force, it may be in the wrong direction. Like, when the beginner wants to push the phaco tip forward he presses over the anterior lip of incision unknowingly and then pushes it forward. (Nasally, if surgeon is sitting on temporal side.) This results in forward movement of the tip but along with that eyeball is also pushed. This creates problems. The operation is done in one part of visual field of microscope. To avoid this it is better not to press at the lips of incision.

The force should be as if the incision is like fulcrum. There is no movement at center of the fulcrum site but both sides move (Fig. 9.10). Another important thing is that there should not be too much pressure on upper or lower lip of incision. Otherwise this may increase the hydration of wound as more fluid comes out. This is because the instrument is not snugly fitting in the incision when we press over the lower lip. This increases the leak from wound. This also decreases the visibility, as we press over the incision the plane of focus of microscope changes.

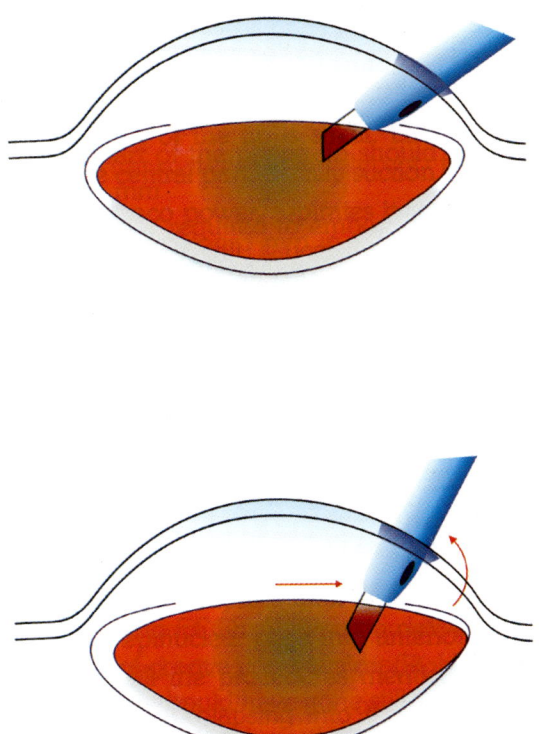

Fig. 9.10: Shows how the incision is used as a fulcrum, after embedding the phaco tip into the nucleus. The movement of the probe should not be like coming out of the anterior chamber

So now it becomes more difficult to operate. In brief, any movement of any instrument, inside the anterior chamber, should be in such a way that you do not press over the wound edges too much. This applies for side port incision and maneuver like rotating the nucleus or chopping should be with minimal stress over the side port incision.

This can be learnt on goats' eyes. This needs practice. All these maneuvers should get stored in action memory (see goat's eye practice).

Similarly, if a phaco beginner wants to push the chopper in the nucleus (of course the nucleus is in firm grip of phaco tip) he may wrongly press over nucleus and at the same time press over the incision. This should be avoided. Pressure should be only at tip and not at side port incision site.

FORCES OTHER THAN VACUUM AND FLOW RATE THAT MODIFY AND HELP IN DOING PHACO

If you want to hold the nucleus and pull it towards the incision, there is a proper way to do this. If you pull it as if you are withdrawing the tip, you will need more vacuum. However, if you move it at incision as a fulcrum, and then push the nucleus towards incision (Fig. 9.11), then, comparatively you need less vacuum, and the nucleus moves easily.

While inserting chopper at capsulorhexis border, if you press it straight then you may dislodge the nucleus from the tip. Whereas, if the same chopper is inserted (use of pointed tip is useful) with force directed towards the tip then it is easy to do chop with less vacuum.

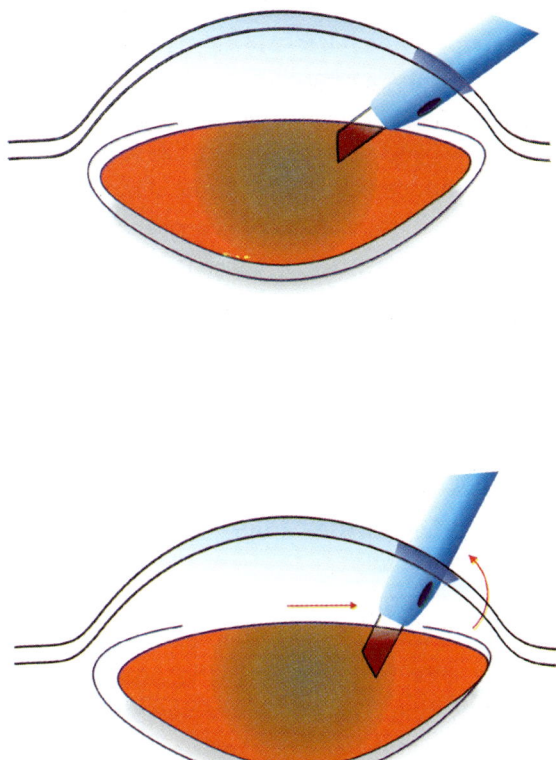

Fig. 9.11: Shows how the nucleus is pulled towards the incision after embedding the phaco tip into the nucleus, using the incision as a fulcrum

When you are dividing the nucleus and the cleavage is incomplete then keeping the phaco tip at the same position, insert the chopper deeper and deeper. You may be afraid of touching the posterior capsule but if you hold the chopper in the manner mentioned above, the sharp point would never touch the capsule. The blunt part, even if touches it, will not rupture the capsule.

The posterior capsule is tough that way and it does not get ruptured easily. In routine ECCE we are afraid of touching posterior capsule, as we know, it may create rent. But in a closed chamber surgery like phaco we need not have this fear. There are more chances of rupturing posterior capsule when it is ballooning forward and has a convex surface. This happens when pressure in anterior chamber is zero and vitreous pressure is more (Fig. 9.12). Great force is required to cause a rent in posterior capsule when it has a concave surface. This is possible when pressure in the anterior chamber is more. This is the reason that while doing all the maneuvers near capsule anterior chamber must be deep.

Polishing posterior capsule with Nightingale ring polisher, though sounds crude, is an easy way. Again you need to take care that you keep the anterior chamber deep while polishing. This makes the capsule concave and as vitreous is pushed behind it will prevent any rent in posterior capsule. This is especially useful when the pupil is not dilated. Polishing capsule with vacuum in undilated pupil is difficult. Alternatively you can polish with low vacuum or even no vacuum. The question, which may arise in your mind, is how can you polish without vacuum? This is possible because pressure in anterior chamber is more than the pressure in aspiration tubing and so fluid moves from anterior chamber to aspiration port due to

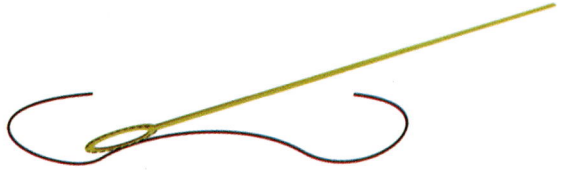

Fig. 9.12: Shows how the ballooning of the posterior capsule occurs in ECCE or shallow anterior chambers

pressure gradient. This movement of fluid will take the lens fibers with it if you rub the handpiece over posterior capsule.

What is the proper way of pushing the chopper in the nucleus?

Imagine that you are holding the nucleus with phaco tip embedded in it and preset vacuum achieved. Now if you wish to insert chopper, lets see how can we do it. Phaco beginner will try to push it as shown in Figure 9.13A. This will create certain problems. If you embed the chopper in a direction opposite to the direction of vacuum force, then there are high chances that it may get dislodged or you need very high vacuum to hold the nucleus. But, if the same embedding is done, as shown in Figure 9.13B, then it supports the vacuum and you need less vacuum to hold the nucleus.

I shall explain in more details about how to embed chopper. The tip of chopper is going inside as if you are feeding the nucleus in the phaco tip. The direction is towards the phaco tip and posterior. The chopper should

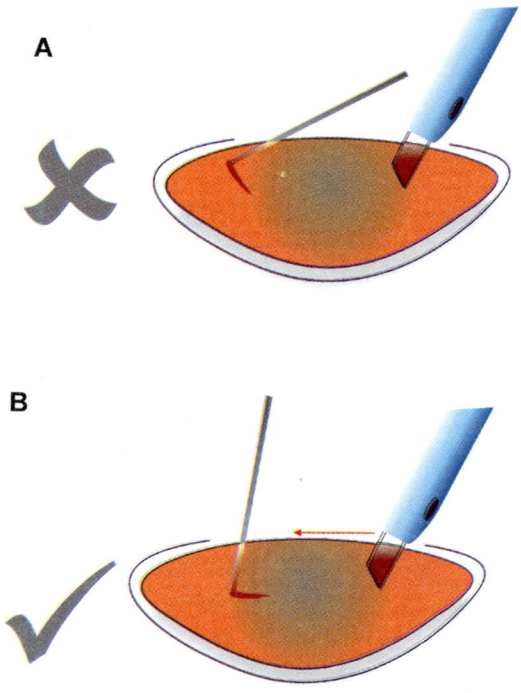

Figs 9.13A and B: A. It is the wrong method of embedding the chopper. **B.** The correct method of embedding the chopper. This will support the vacuum and comparatively less vacuum is required to crack the nucleus

go deep enough, at least 1.5 mm. (When this happens, the small part of the bent portion of chopper will also get embedded in the soft nucleus.) This way we are supporting the vacuum while embedding the chopper. You need lesser vacuum to hold the nucleus and chopping becomes easy.

With phaco tip embedded what should be the proper way of moving the nucleus towards the incision site?
Once the phaco tip is embedded for chopping or Woodcutter's technique, it is always better to move the nucleus towards incision site. To achieve this you have to move along the force of the vacuum otherwise the nucleus may get released from the tip. Move it as if you are pushing towards incision with the tip, making the probe more vertical (Fig. 9.14).

How to avoid kinking of the irrigation tubing near the phaco handpiece junction?
For this, use harder sleeve over the irrigation tube. This does not allow the irrigation tube to be kinked. Kinking is a great problem, as that will cause sudden collapse of chamber that has its own disadvantages (Fig. 9.15).

Phaco for beginners and different mistakes which are done in learning phase

Many mistakes occur knowingly or unknowingly while doing phaco in initial stages. I would like to elaborate few common mistakes, which occur in initial stages.

Side port—While doing side port, if more pressure is given, and the entry with 20 gauge needle in the anterior chamber occurs uncontrolled, then sometimes there are chances of iridodialysis or trauma to the iris or anterior capsule.

If this extension in anterior capsule is too far towards the periphery and you are not able to do a complete

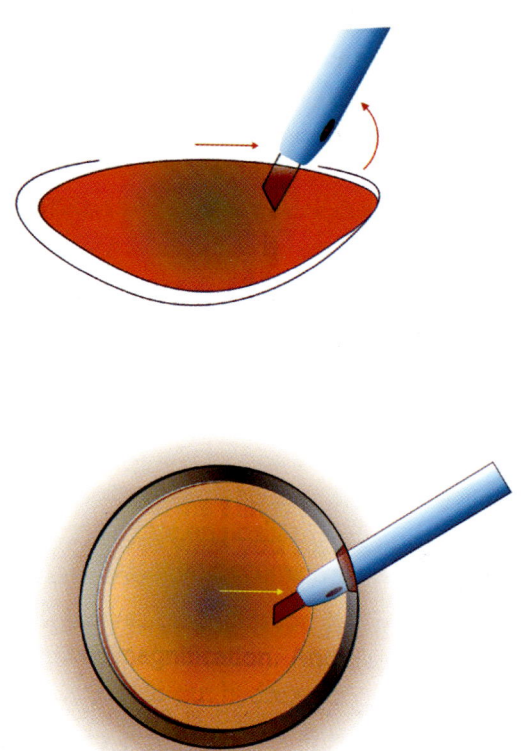

Fig. 9.14: Shows how the position of the probe is, i.e. 70 to 80 degrees vertical, and not horizontal

capsulorhexis, then you may have to convert canopener capsulorhexis and to ECCE.

If the side port tunnel width becomes too large or **very** small then it may leak during phaco and may cause surge.

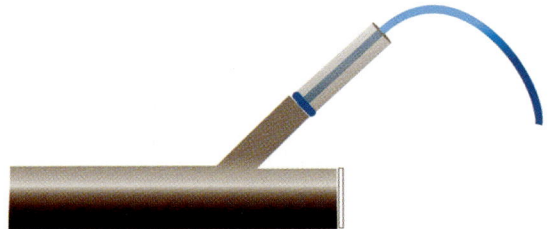

Fig. 9.15: Shows the use of harder sleeve over the irrigation tube to avoid the kinking of the tube

In such cases it should be sutured. Make another fresh side port.

Sometimes the side port may go more corneal and into the layers of cornea. This makes maneuvering in the chamber difficult. The hydration of the side port occurs more if the width of incision is more. It is better to make another side port near this.

Main incision: The most common mistake to occur here is, we go more limbal and this causes iris prolapse. Also one should not go more in the layers of cornea. This makes the tunnel width more. Then the maneuvering in the chamber becomes difficult.

If the main incision becomes larger, it leaks and may cause surge. In problematic incision suture the incision and make fresh incision at approachable site.

While maneuvering the instruments you should not press over the lips of the incisions. The fluid will leak and the anterior chamber becomes shallow repeatedly. Do not press over the incision while maneuvering in the chamber. Sometimes the eyeball moves nasally while operating from temporal side. This is because the phaco tip presses over the lip and rotates the eye. Instead move the tip inside without pressing over the lips of incision. Also you should avoid touching the iris as this may also constrict the pupil.

Deep anterior chamber is must throughout the procedure. The advantage of deep anterior chamber is that you get more space for maneuvering the instruments. Also while doing capsulorhexis, if the anterior chamber remains deep, the chances of extension of capsulorhexis to the periphery are less. There are less chances of rent in posterior capsule. It is easier to polish the posterior capsule if the anterior chamber is deep, because the posterior capsule will have a concave surface.

I am learning phaco under topical. During surgery I feel I am not comfortable with topical. I want to convert to peribulbar block. How can I convert?

If you feel the pressure is high from behind, but there is no expulsive hemorrhage, then push viscoelastics in eye. The incisions are self sealing. Then give peribulbar block. If necessary, you can close eyelids and give massage over the closed lids to cause hypotony.

Anterior chamber is getting collapsed and visco-elastic is coming out repeatedly. What should I do?

Rule out pressure of speculum or any other thing on eyeball. The tunnel width may be very less. So it does not act as a self sealing incision. In such cases use other hydroxypropyl methylcellulose, which is more viscous.

Even then if the anterior chamber is becoming shallower, then your incision may be improper. Close the incision and make another tunnel.

Sometimes the peribulbar block, if given helps, give massage with closed eyelid, of course after closing the incision. Again you can proceed further after you get the desired hypotony.

If iris is coming out through incision repeatedly, what should I do?

Insert a small repositor from the side port and try to reposit it back. Never try to reposit the prolapsing iris from main incision itself, as it will again prolapse immediately. Thus, unnecessarily you are causing trauma to the iris and even wasting your time. Alternatively you can inject visco from side port and try to reposit the iris. Sometimes you may have to close the incision and make a new incision, which is more corneal. So no iris prolapse occurs. Another alternative is to apply the iris retractors if iris is floppy.

If iris is repeatedly getting in phaco tip

If the iris is floppy then it gets attracted towards the probe and even may come into the probe. Usually the iris becomes more floppy if it has come into the probe even once. This is called iris chaffing. This occurs most commonly in cases of semidilated pupil. In such cases avoid that area of floppy iris and do phaco in other area. But even then it keeps on coming into the probe. Then best possible, which can be done, is to apply iris retractors and then proceed further.

Chapter 10

Subluxated Lens, Small Pupil and Pediatric Cataract

Subluxated Lens

It is difficult to do the phaco in subluxated lens as the pressure differences in anterior chamber which occur during the phaco, cause movment of the lens, which may tear the zonules, enhancing the subluxation. The function of aspiration flow rate is to attract the loose fragments. As the lens itself is loose here, it gets attracted towards aspiration port exaggerating the existing problems. Now you will be able to understand that the basic principle, while managing a case of subluxated lens, is to prevent sudden changes in anterior chamber pressure. Similarly, sudden collapse of anterior chamber after removing the phaco tip will also cause more problems. To avoid this following steps are taken:

1. Choose the site of main phaco incision in the area opposite to the subluxated part.
2. Take side port incision accordingly. Take care, not to allow the anterior chamber to collapse. If it starts collapsing inject hydroxypropyl methylcellulose.
3. Make main phaco incision taking care not to allow the collapse of chamber. If it occurs inject methylcellulose from side port.
4. Use of Trypan blue definitely helps in demarcating capsulorhexis border in immature cataract too. But you need to be careful for it may go beyond through subluxted part and stain the posterior capsule. This decreases the red glow intensity and hampers the visibility.

5. While doing capsulorhexis anterior chamber should be deep. But, using too much of viscoelastics will push the lens far more posteriorly. Hence, it is necessary to use only appropriate amount of viscoelastics.

6. Start doing the capsulorhexis in the part where the zonules are tough. In the part where zonules are weak capsulorhexis has a tendency to extend towards periphery. Try to stabilize the nucleus by supporting it with a dialer or blunt spatula from side port and continue with capsulorhexis.

7. Once the capsulorhexis is complete insert the endocapsular ring (capsular tension ring). While inserting the endocapsular ring, take care that zonular dehiscence will not occur.

8. Push the endocapsular ring through main phaco incision. Then support it by dialer from side port so that it does not stretch the capsulorhexis (Fig. 10.1). Depth of the anterior chamber should be maintained throughout the procedure. It should not be too deep or too shallow. The trailing end of endocapsular ring is pushed with Mcpherson forceps. If, with this, it does not go in the bag then dial with the dialer in the bag. This is necessary because, if the loop goes in the angle it becomes difficult to dial it inside the capsular bag. If the trailing end goes in angle of anterior chamber then pull the endocapsular ring with dialer (from side port) from the part which is near the capsular rim. Then with other dialer (from

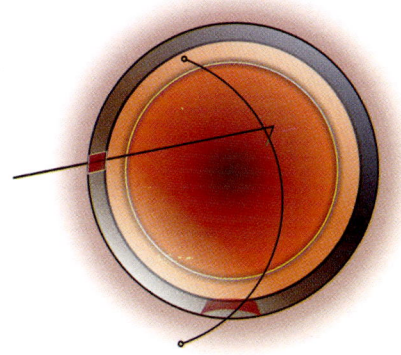

Fig. 10.1: Shows how the dialer from the side port
supports the endocapsular ring

main phaco incision) engage the eyelet of the
endocapsular ring. Then slide the eyelet of the ring
in the bag. If it is not getting dislodged then the dialer
from side port will help in dislodging.

9. Once the endocapsular ring is inside, then we can
do phaco with lower preset vacuum and lower flow
rate as less turbulence is expected in anterior
chamber.

10. Do not do any maneuver, which will pull the nucleus
in the axis of weak zonules.

11. Do not allow the chamber to collapse when you
remove the phaco tip. Before that inject
hydroxypropyl methylcellulose from side port. This
will not allow the anterior chamber to collapse.

12. In irrigation aspiration, use less vacuum and less flow
rate.

13. If vitreous prolapses and comes out through the side port and if it does not interfere with the maneuvers, there is no need to do vitrectomy at this stage. Do phaco, do irrigation and aspiration of cortex, put intraocular lens and then it is time to do vitrectomy. The vitreous strands that come out through side port actually support the capsule bag during maneuver. When this happens it is better to put intraocular lens of 6.5 mm diameter and above the anterior capsule.

14. If vitreous prolapse is more and comes out through main incision it is wise to remove the lens capsule, lens nucleus and cortex and then put anterior chamber lens or Daljit Singh's iris claw lens.

15. Whenever intraocular lens is to be put, choose the one with a larger diameter; so that slight decentration of lens will not create any problem. It should be done so that there is least stretch on zonules. If vitrectomy is done then put intraocular lens on the anterior surface of capsule.

16. Ensure that the wound is leak proof at the end of surgery and there are no vitreous strands in anterior chamber. Intraocular lens should be well centered.

SMALL PUPIL

Causes

- Pseudoexfoliation
- Posterior synechiae
- Inflamed eye
- Complicated cataract

- Pilocarpinised pupil
- If dilated initially on same day then the pupil does not dilate again.

Mechanism of Dilating and Method of Dilatation

1. Peribulbar block; by blocking ciliary ganglion
2. Subtenon Xylocaine; by local absorption
3. Intracameral Xylocaine 0.5% preservative free; by locally acting on muscles
4. Intracameral Epitrate; by locally acting on dilator pupillae muscles
5. Iris Retractors (Nylon hook with adjustable silicon retaining sleeve
6. Viscoelastics, healon, mechanical dilatation.

Continuous Curvilinear Capsulorhexis => No special precaution is required if iris retractors are applied.

If iris retractors are not applied and the size of pupil is around 4 mm, then, pupillary margin acts as a fulcrum and a regular midperipheral rhexis of about 5 to 5.5 mm can be performed easily.

You can try cycloplegics like cyclopentolate and epinephrine

If you are operating under topical then it is always better to shift over to peribulbar block. This is not to relieve the pain but this helps in dilating the pupil through of ciliary ganglion block.

Subconjunctival Xylocaine with adrenaline (unless contraindicated) if spread all around, will dilate the pupil.

All incisions on cornea should be little more inside the limbus (specially the entry in anterior chamber), so that iris does not prolapse through these incisions.

Use of intracameral epinephrine may help.

Use of adrenaline in Balanced Salt Solution is one way.

Break the posterior synechiae if there are any. Do not tear the capsule. Try to remain on iris side.

If nothing helps then retract iris with use iris retractors.

How to make incisions for introducing iris retractors?

This is done in the same way as side port incision. While doing the side port incisions for iris retractors, be careful that these side ports are at limbus and not clear corneal. If this side port is made clear corneal, then iris (about 1 to 1.5 mm) is not retracted fully. These are four in number in addition to the existing side port incision.

The incision for iris retractors should be one on each side of main phaco incision. This helps in avoiding the iris coming in the way of introduction of phaco tip. The other two iris retractor incisions should be diagonally opposite direction. The ideal sites for iris retractors are said to be at 10.30, 1.30, 4.30 and 7.30 o'clock position (Fig. 10.2). So a perfect square occurs in the center. Introduce the iris retractor through the 1 mm incision, hook/engage the iris and pull the iris retractor and then fix it by the silicon sleeve. Take care that the iris retractor does not tear the anterior capsule.

The advantage of iris retractor is that the phaco surgery is possible without any change in routine surgical steps

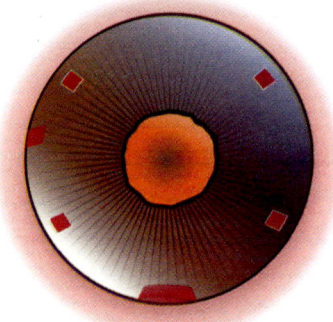

Fig. 10.2: Shows the approximate positions of incisions of the iris retractors, the side port and the main incision

once the iris retractor is in place. The synechiae can be easily tackled. The iris does not come in the phaco tip. Postoperatively the pupil remains round.

If we stretch the iris by iris manipulators or dialer, then the iris becomes floppy and repeatedly it gets attracted to the phaco tip. So I think it is not good to dilate pupil by this way for phaco technique.

PEDIATRIC CATARACT

This type of cataract is little different from routine senile cataracts. Here we have to take some additional precautions in managing these types of cataracts. Here, also, I will like to mention some practical tips instead of mentioning the whole theoretical part, with which all of you are well versed.

In first step the incision should be small than routine phaco incision. Usually make about 2.0 mm. It should be clear corneal. The advantage is that iris adhesion is not there and prolapse of iris is also not there. It is always better to avoid touching the iris, so inflammation induced is less. Secondly, when we make small incision the viscoelastic does not come out easily. Use Inamura-Utrata forceps for capsulorhexis. This goes through small incision. Use trypan blue. This helps a lot, specially when we do posterior capsulorhexis. It differentiates the anterior and posterior openings in the capsule.

Try to make small capsulorhexis. In pediatric cases the capsule is elastic. So it extends towards periphery.

Once the capsulorhexis is complete then aspirate the contents with small irrigation aspiration cannula like Simcoe. You can enlarge the incision but a smaller incision is helpful in maintaining the anterior chamber.

If the patient is *less than six years* then it is better to perform posterior capsulorhexis with Utrata-Tnamura capsulorhexis forceps.

Usually 3 to 3.5 mm posterior capsulorhexis is performed. The posterior capsule in these patients is very thin. Hence, avoid doing larger rhexis than this. Also the IOL may be done through the posterior capsulorhexis if the posterior capsulorhexis is large. After completing the posterior capsulorhexis, if patient is below one year, then it is better to perform anterior vitrectomy. All this avoids opacification behind IOL. The PCIOL is implanted in the bag. The optic of the IOL is passed below the posterior capsulorhexis keeping the haptics in capsular bag. This is called *optic capture*.

Plenty of steroids should be given intra-as well as post-operatively, both locally as well as systemically with good antibiotic cover. The patients are called for regular follow-ups. In initial days the follow-up is more frequent.

Our Contributions to Ophthalmology

Appendix I

RECTAL MUCOUS MEMBRANE GRAFT IN DRY EYE

In dry eye, due to S J syndrome and chemical burn, the main problem is destruction of conjunctiva. There is extensive conjunctival damage resulting mainly in deficiency of the mucin component of tear film, which is secreted by the goblet cells of the conjunctiva. The conjunctiva contains goblet cells. This results in mucin deficiency dry eye. So the ideal way of treating this will be replacing the goblet cells. To replace these goblet cells, I do rectal mucous membrane graft in these patients. Why to use rectal mucous membrane only? Because, it is studded with goblet cells. The buccal mucous membrane does not contain goblet cells. So even if you transplant it, that serves the purpose of mucous membrane but does not replace the goblet cells. If we use the rectal mucous membrane of the patient then that replaces the goblet cells too. This becomes the natural continuous source of mucin.

In this procedure rectal mucous membrane of the patient is obtained with the help of general surgeon. Patient is operated under spinal anesthesia. The mucous membrane is obtained from posterior wall of rectum. Nearly 30 mm × 60 mm is sufficient for both eyes and both fornices. This mucous membrane is kept in povidone-

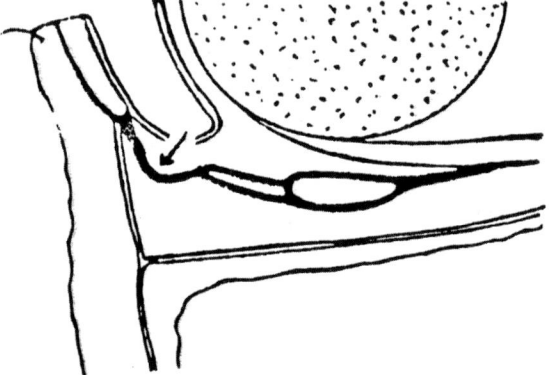

Step 1: Lower fornix conjunctiva incised

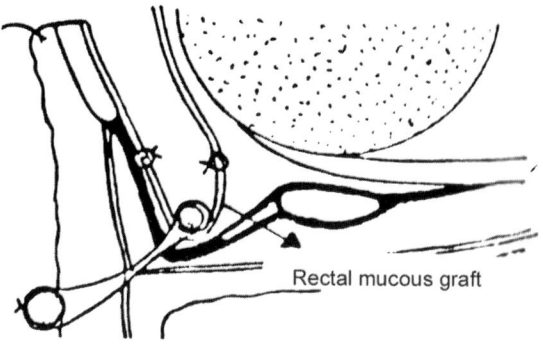

Step 2: Lower fornix deepening suture
holding rectal mucous graft

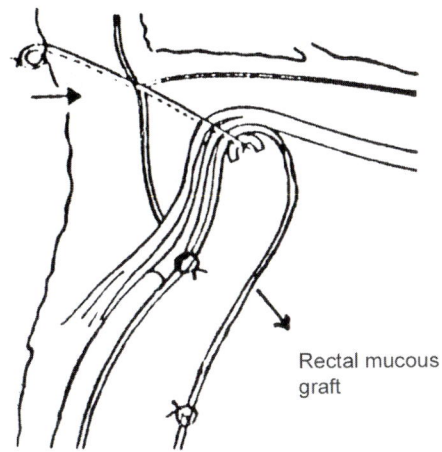

Rectal mucous
graft

Step 3: Upper fornix deepening suture
holding rectal mucous graft

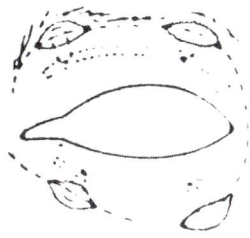

Step 4: External appearance after completion of surgery

Fig. I.1: Steps of surgery

iodine solution 0.5%, which is used for cleansing mucous membrane for 30 minutes.

The conjunctiva is incised in lower and upper fornix. No part of conjunctiva is excised. To the free edges of conjunctiva the rectal mucous membrane of 30 mm × 15 mm is sutured (Fig. I.1). Fornix deepening sutures are taken (as in any other shallow fornix repair surgery refer to J.R.O. Collin systematic eyelid surgery). The surgery is same as any other fornix deepening surgery but instead of buccal mucous membrane use rectal mucous membrane. There is no need of any shell to be put.

This gives continuous source of mucin. The results of this procedure are quite encouraging. Of course the other surgeries may be needed like stem cell graft and keratoplasty.

Frequently Asked Questions:

It must have high chances of infection?
Really speaking, no! The mucous membrane really has great resistance against infection. This is some thing similar to buccal mucous membrane graft. The buccal mucous membrane also has high bacterial flora. But it does not cause infection in the eye and the oral wound also gets healed up without infection.

Appendix II

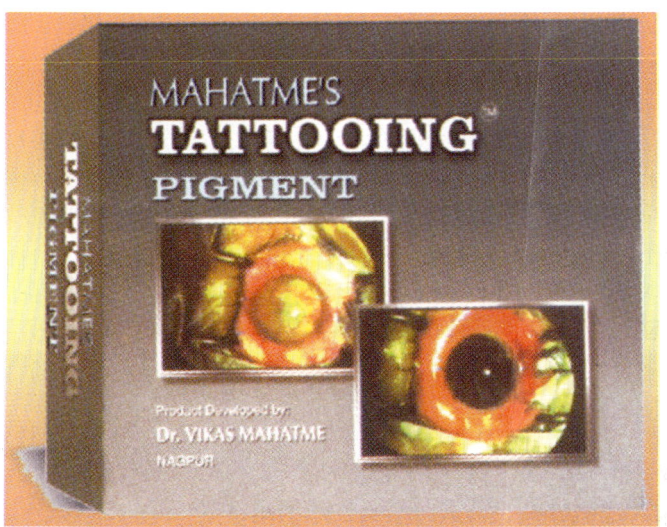

NEW PIGMENT FOR COSMETIC CORNEAL TATTOOING

Tattooing was known and practiced long before the Christian era. In primitive civilizations, tattooing distinguished men of rank and status. Tattooing of the cornea for unsightly leucomas is of ancient lineage.

In the practice of Ophthalmology it is not always that you can give vision to a patient. There are occasions when you have to add a cosmetic value to the patient's life, like in blind eye with corneal opacity. Simple answer is tattooing. Then why tattooing is not done by general ophthalmologists? There are two main reasons. Firstly, there is non-availability of chemical pigment and secondly, whatever pigments are used for tattooing are irritants for eye. Eye doesn't remain quiet after the procedure and corneal epithelium doesn't remain stable on the pigment. The ideal pigment or dye used for tattooing should be inert and easily available. On this background, I wish to draw your attention to a new pigment for tattooing. It is not water-soluble nor lipid soluble. I tried it initially on blind eyes and that too, in those patients who were prepared to get their eyes enucleated afterwards. Next, I tried the pigment in-patients of corneal opacity. The results are satisfactory beyond expectations.

For different types of opacities different surgical techniques are used.

1. **Multiple needle puncture:** This technique is used for superficial opacities which are not dense (nebular to macular grade). This procedure involves spreading the pigment which is in the powder form over the opacity. Multiple needle punctures are done in such a way that the pigment will go inside but there will not be any corneal perforation. In brief, strokes should be oblique, made into different directions, and should not penetrate deeper to superficial one-third of stroma. Wash the pigment with saline. See extent of opacity, which is still remaining. If some part of opacity is still

visible then spread the pigment and repeat the procedure till you are satisfied. Please keep it in mind that under microscope the opacity may be visible but in daylight it may be acceptable cosmetically (Fig. II.1).

2. **Lamellar resection:** If opacity is dense and superficial cornea is transparent or translucent, this method is used.

Make an incision 3 mm in width and nearly one-third thickness of cornea at one of the edges of opacity. A lamellar resection was done separating superficial cornea from the deep cornea with the help of crescent blade. Injection Hyaluronidase 150 I.U. in 2 ml is injected. This helps to create a proper plane of cleavage, as it is difficult to create plane of cleavage in the scarred tissue. Once the Hyaluronidase is injected then separation is easy with blunt instrument like curved iris repositor. After this the pigment is spread between the superficial and deep corneal lamellae. The incision can be sutured with 9 zero nylon (Fig. II.2).

3. **Lamellar graft:** When the opacity is dense and superficial then following procedure is adopted.

Scrape off the corneal epithelium over the opacity. If the corneal opacity is involving full diameter of cornea, make a partial thickness incision in circular fashion so as to separate the stem cells and conjunctiva. Then take the lamellar graft of one-third of the corneal thickness from glycerol preserved cornea. Tuck this graft below the stem cells and conjunctiva. If the opacity

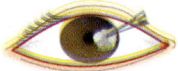

Fig. II.1: Multiple needle puncture

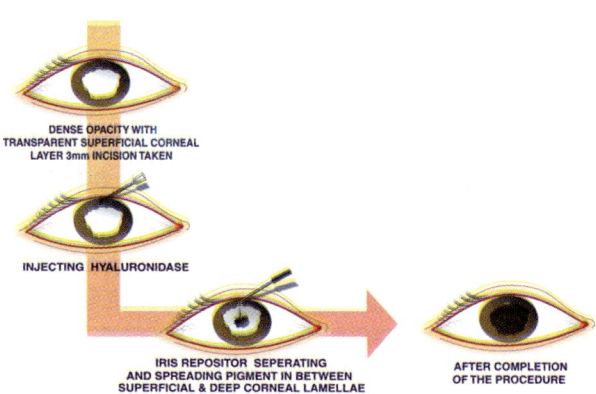

DENSE OPACITY WITH
TRANSPARENT SUPERFICIAL CORNEAL
LAYER 3mm INCISION TAKEN

INJECTING HYALURONIDASE

IRIS REPOSITOR SEPERATING
AND SPREADING PIGMENT IN BETWEEN
SUPERFICIAL & DEEP CORNEAL LAMELLAE

AFTER COMPLETION
OF THE PROCEDURE

Fig. II.2: Lamellar resection

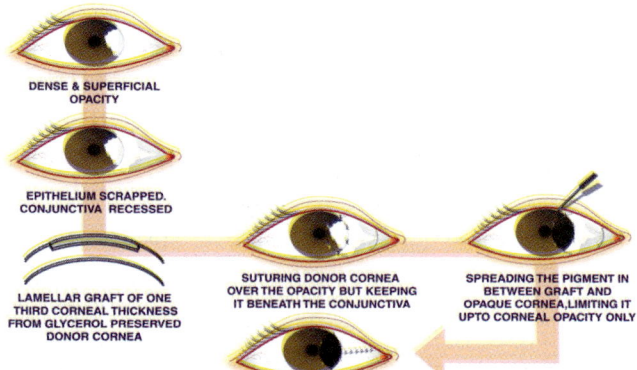

DENSE & SUPERFICIAL
OPACITY

EPITHELIUM SCRAPPED.
CONJUNCTIVA RECESSED

LAMELLAR GRAFT OF ONE
THIRD CORNEAL THICKNESS
FROM GLYCEROL PRESERVED
DONOR CORNEA

SUTURING DONOR CORNEA
OVER THE OPACITY BUT KEEPING
IT BENEATH THE CONJUNCTIVA

SPREADING THE PIGMENT IN
BETWEEN GRAFT AND
OPAQUE CORNEA,LIMITING IT
UPTO CORNEAL OPACITY ONLY

RECESSED CONJUNCTIVA SUTURED IN ITS PLACE

Fig. II.3: Lamellar graft

is small size but dense and superficial then tuck the graft like in epikeratophakia. Once this is done, suture the graft with continuous 9 zero nylon. But before tying the knot the pigment is spread below the graft and then suture is tied (Fig. II.3).

4. **Procedure for opacity of mixed variety**: For example central dense deep opacity with peripheral nebular superficial, then combination of procedures can be adopted. Central area is done by lamellar resection while the peripheral faint opacity is done by multiple needle punctures.

Areas that Deserve Improvements

The color of pigment is dark black and so may not match with blue iris of other eye.

The color fades after 5-6 years but does not altogether vanish.

Advantage: The greatest advantage is that the pigment does not cause any irritation.

About the EASY BREATH — An Asset for Ophthalmic Surgery

This gadget (Fig. II.4) is an asset for ophthalmic surgery that allows patient to breath freely during surgery. Most of the patients in our country are from village area. Also most of the patients getting operated for cataract surgery are old aged. These patients are afraid of surgery and if their face is covered by drape they feel too much

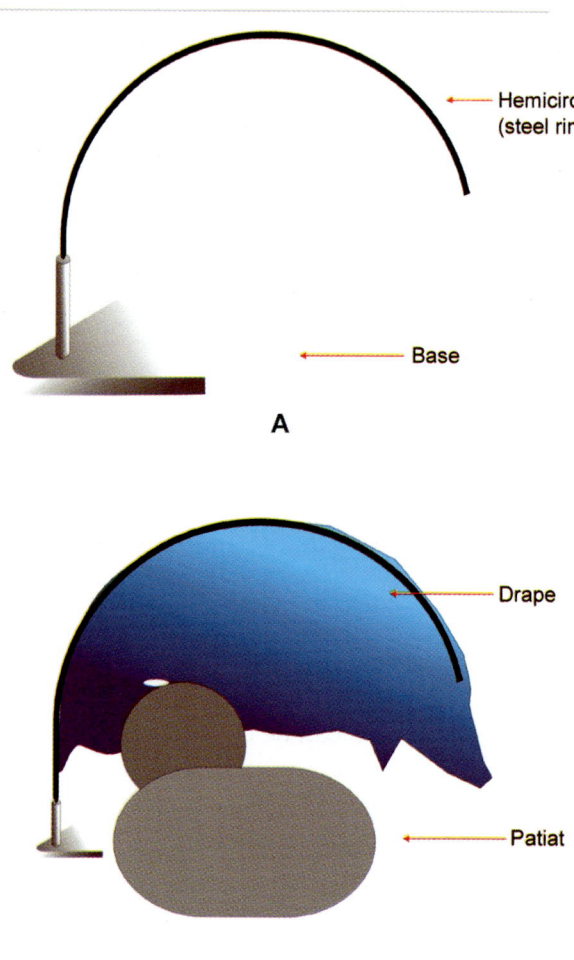

Fig. II.4: Easy breath

suffocated. Easy breath really helps patient to breathe easily by giving more room. The drapes do not fall on nose of the patient. In urban area operation theater is airconditioned. In developed countries, they use oxygen tubings near nose. So patient does not feel suffocation. All the surgeries are attended by anesthetist but in rural area we may not have all these facilities. So in this case easy breathe can be a boon. This can be carried to the camps too. It has got a heavy base on which a small hemicircle arm rests. In spite of this if patient feels suffocated and his spO2 starts falling down, we can place an oxygen tube in the space. In brief it avoids claustrophobia (fear of getting suffocated).

Advantages:
- Space required to place the easy breath is less.
- It provides enough room for giving nasal oxygen if necessary.
- Patient's level of co-operation increases.
- It is economical also.
- Ring and the base can be sterilized.
- It can be carried for camps too.

Appendix III

> WHAT WE ARE BORN IS GOD'S GIFT TO US
>
> WHAT WE BECOME IS OUR GIFT TO GOD

SCLERAL FLAP ELEVATION BY FILTRATION ENHANCING KNOT IN TRABECULECTOMY

The basic problem in trabeculectomy operation or any filtration operation is that filtration is maximum on day one and gradually as wound heals up, filtration becomes less.

At this time our expectations are that we should achieve target pressure. Naturally we want to keep IOP below target pressure for first few days. So that, even if wound heals and filtration becomes less we get appropriate target pressure on long term. But in getting this, sometimes we land up in a problem of flat anterior chamber and its consequences.

To avoid this it would be better if we aim at IOP slightly higher than target pressure for first few days and then reduce it as per our requirement by enhancing filtration. But, how to do this? For this I have come out with this new technique.

To overcome this problem of flat AC, filtration-enhancing knot can be of great help. We can keep IOP above target pressure in the initial postoperative period and filtration can be enhanced thereafter as per requirement, simply by elevating scleral flap, holding the filtration enhancing knot. As the IOP is above target pressure on day one without any hesitation patient can be discharged on same day. Secondly, if IOP is maintained for first few days and then after seven days if pressure is reduced to great extent like 4 mm of Hg then cornea is sucked in rather than iris lens diaphragm being pushed forward. This happens because once the anatomy is restored and maintained then even if IOP falls to zero probability of flat anterior chamber is less. We will get sucking of cornea in. But the iris lens diaphragm is not pushed forward.

Procedure

Limbal based conjunctival flap is made (Fig. III.1). Then routine trabeculectomy surgery is done. After excising the deep scleral flap and before suturing superficial scleral flap, take 8-0 nylon suture. This is passed through conjunctiva one mm away from limbus and in the region of center of superficial conjunctiva flap, then through tenons, then partial thickness of scleral flap and out through tenons and conjunctiva (Fig. III.2). A loose knot is tied on conjunctiva (Fig. III.3). This I call it as filtration-enhancing knot. Then trabeculectomy wound closure is done in usual fashion (Fig. III.4) aiming postoperative pressure slightly higher than the target pressure. After 4 days the IOP is measured. If bleb is small then filtration-enhancing knot

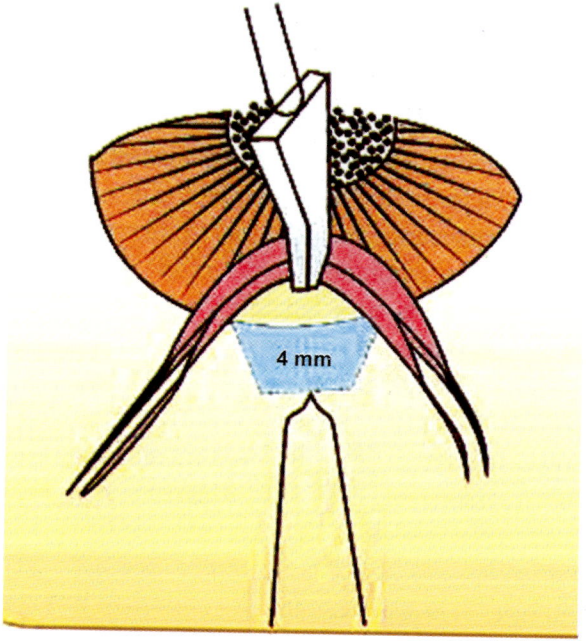

Fig. III.1: Limbal based conjunctival flap

is pulled up. This elevates the scleral flap and conjunctiva, which will cause aqueous to leak below conjunctiva and will be visible as bleb. This should be done under topical anesthesia on slit lamp or operating microscope. Every fourth day patient is called till the IOP is below target pressure and bleb is good for consecutive three visits. If it is not, then by pulling the filtration-enhancing knot bleb can be increased. Suturolysis or digital massage can be combined if necessary. Usually the suture taken through

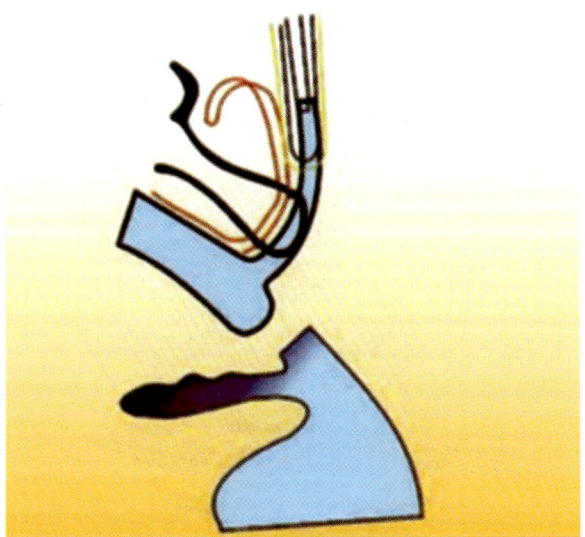

Fig. III.2: 8°-Nylon suture passed through conjunctiva, Tenon's capsule superficial scleral flap, Tenon's and conjunctiva

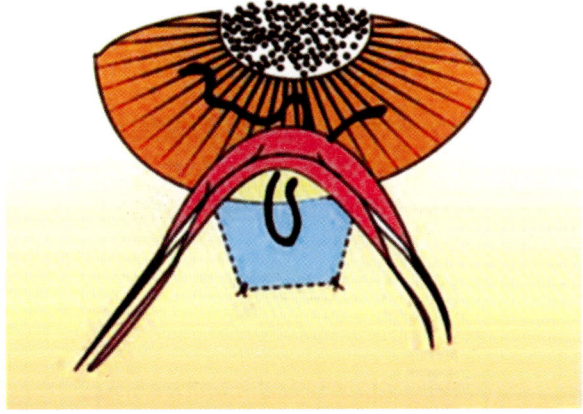

Fig. III.3: See how the suture looks after scleral flap is sutured

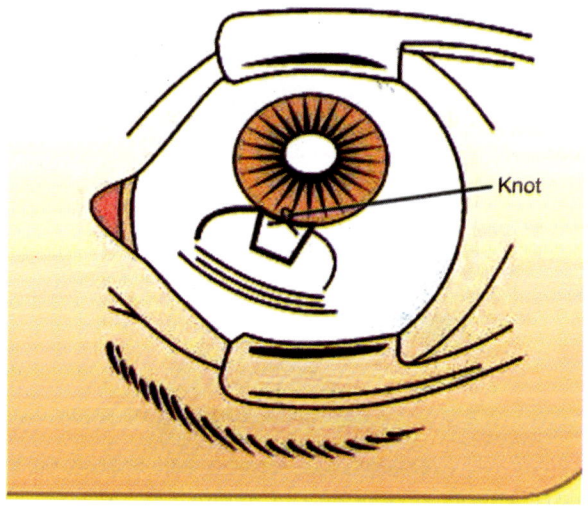

Fig. III.4: Sutured knot seen above conjunctiva

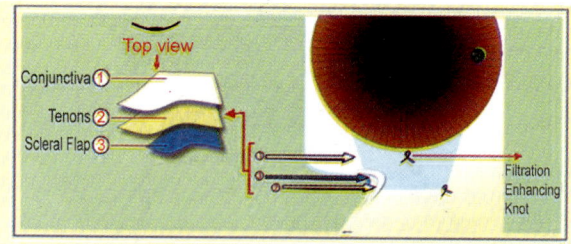

Fig. III.5: Top view—filtration enhancing knot

superficial scleral flap (8 zero nylon of filtration-enhancing knot) is removed after one month.

Area of Added Attention and Possible Problems

- Filtration-enhancing knot suture should pass through tenons.
- It may cause foreign body sensation. Pulling may cause small hemorrhage. Rarely leak may be there from the suture area. This can be prevented if needle passes through tenons and partial thickness of sclera.

Bibliography

1. Comparison of Conventional Chop technique with Wood-cutters nucleus cracking technique. Presented at AIOS, Varanasi, Jan 2004. By Dr. Seema Dharmadhikari.
2. Dada VK: Fun with phaco.
3. Hard Nuclei? No problem!" Poster Presentation at ICO, Sydney, Australia, April 2002.
4. Jaffe NS, Jaffe MS, Jaffe GF: Cataract Surgery and its Complications, Sixth edition.
5. Kelman CD: Phacoemulsification and aspiration. *Am J Ophthalmol* **64:**23-35, 1967.
6. Mehta KR, Alpar JJ: The Art of Phacoemulsification.
7. Newer technique makes Nuclear Fragmentation by Phaco Easy: A comparative study in same eye. Presented at AIOS, Calcutta, Jan 2001.
8. Paul Koch: Stop and Chop. Mastering Phacoemulsification Thorofare, NJ: SLACK Inc, 1993.
9. Prospective Study Comparing Nuclear Division by Chop Technique and Woodcutters Nucleus Cracking Technique (Newer technique) in Phacoemulsification presented at DOC. Nurnberg, Germany (14th Annual meeting of German Ophthalmic Surgeons and International Symposium) April 2001.
10. Rectal mucous membrane graft in dry eye. Indian Journal of Ophthalmology, Vol.47, No. 2, June 99, 129-32.
11. Sachdev M: Phacoemulsification—Practical Guide.
12. Seibel BS: Phacodynamics—Mastering the Tools and Techniques of Phacoemulsification Surgery, Second edition.
13. Steinert RF: Cataract Surgery—Technique, Complications, Management. Second edition.
14. Surge: No more a problem with modified phaco sleeve. By Dr. Seema Dharmadhikari. Presented at AIOS, New Delhi, Feb 2003.
15. Woodcutters split hard nuclei at ease. Presented at Rome Symposium April 2001.

MAHATME EYE BANK AND EYE HOSPITAL
(Recognised Institute for Postgraduation)
Nagpur and Mumbai, India

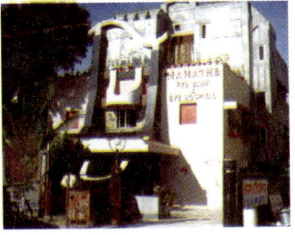

N A G P U R

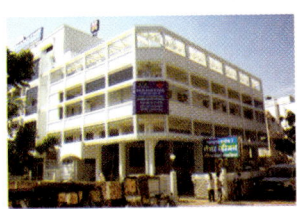

**Main Hospital
Nagpur**

**Branch Hospital
Somalwada, Nagpur**

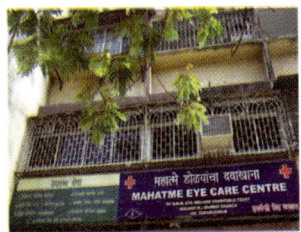

M U M B A I

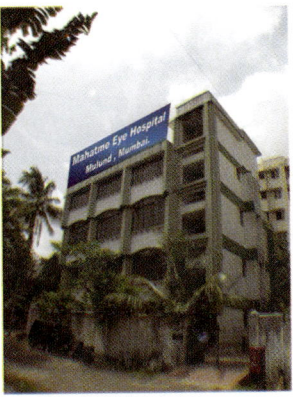

**Mahatme Eye Care
Centre, Mulund, Mumbai**

**Mahatme Eye Hospital
Mulund, Mumbai**

contact@mahatmehospital.com

Learning   Opportunities

- Short term hands on phaco training program.
- Postgraduate courses in ophthalmology DNB (Diplomate of National Board, Government of India recognised); DOMS (recognised by CPS).
- Examination center for ICO (International Council of Ophthalmology) Assessment.
- Phaco training center, recognised by ICO.
- Post MS/DNB/DO resident fellowship in Phaco and General Ophthalmology.
- B. Optometry and D. Optometry courses after 12th Std.
- Ophthalmic Technician and Hospital Assistant Courses for 10th and 12th passed students.
- Certificate course in Computer Application and Hospital Assistant.

The Institute can make available for you—

- **Pigment for Corneal Tattooing:** Marketed by M/s. Appasmy Associates.
- **Cornea**: For optical and therapeutic keratoplasty, on request.
- **Ocular Creative Craft**: A CD on compilation of Surgical Skills including woodcutter's nucleus cracking technique (Surgeon: Dr. Vikas Mahatme) Marketed by M/s. S.V. Creations.
- **Easy breath:** An asset for ophthalmic surgery; permits free air entry and avoids falling of drapes over patients face.
- **Eye soft:** Hospital management software for ophthal-mologist.

MAHATME EYE BANK AND EYE HOSPITAL
Main Hospital

16, Central Excise Colony, Ring Road,
Chatrapati Square, Wardha Road,
Nagpur-440 015, Maharashtra
India

e-mail	:	vikas@mahatmehospital.com
e-mail	:	vikasmahatme@rediffmail.com
e-mail	:	contact@mahatmehospital.com
Web	:	www.mahatmehospital.com
Fax	:	0091-712-2242202
Phone	:	0091-712-2222556, 2234345

Branch Hospital

2163-C Chintaman Nagar, Somalwada,
Near Rajiv Nagar, Nagpur
Tel: 0712-2289101 to 106

Mumbai Branch

102-B, Varadlaxmi, Gokhle Road
Near Jai Ganesh Cinema
Mulund-East, Mumbai-81
Tel: 0091-22-25657090
e-mail:
mulundbr@mahatmehospital.com
meccmmb@rediffmail.com

Index